Teach Yourself VISUALLY™
Yoga

Visual

From
maranGraphics®

&

Wiley Publishing, Inc.

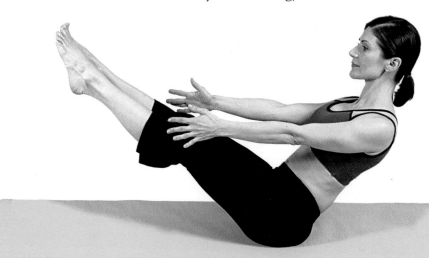

Teach Yourself VISUALLY™ Yoga

Published by
Wiley Publishing, Inc.
909 Third Avenue
New York, NY 10022

Published simultaneously in Canada

Copyright © 2003 by maranGraphics Inc.
5755 Coopers Avenue
Mississauga, Ontario, Canada
L4Z 1R9

Library of Congress Control Number:

ISBN: 0-7645-2580-8

Manufactured in the United States of America

10 9 8 7 6 5 4 3 2 1

1K/QR/QV/QT/MG

Trademark Acknowledgments

Important Numbers

For U.S. corporate orders, please call maranGraphics at 800-469-6616 or fax 905-890-9434.

For general information on our products and services, please contact our Customer Care Department within the U.S. at 800-762-2974, outside the U.S. at 317-572-3993 or fax 317-572-4002.

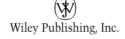

Wiley Publishing, Inc.   is a trademark of Wiley Publishing, Inc.

U.S. Corporate Sales	U.S. Trade Sales
Contact maranGraphics at (800) 469-6616 or fax (905) 890-9434.	Contact Wiley at (800) 762-2974 or fax (317) 572-4002.

VISUAL TESTIMONIALS

"I write to extend my
thanks and appreciation
for your books.
They are clear, easy to follow,
and straight to the point.
Keep up the good work!
I bought several of your books
and they are just right!
No regrets! I will always
buy your books because
they are the best."

**Seward Kollie
Dakar, Senegal**

"I just had to let you and
your company know how
great I think your books are.
I just purchased my third
Visual book (my first two
are dog-eared now!) and,
once again, your product has
surpassed my expectations.
The expertise, thought, and
effort that go into each book
are obvious, and I sincerely
appreciate your efforts.
Keep up the wonderful work!"

**Tracey Moore
Memphis, TN**

"I am an avid fan of
your Visual books.
If I need to learn anything,
I just buy one of your books and
learn the topic in no time.
Wonders! I have even trained
my friends to give me
Visual books as gifts."

**Illona Bergstrom
Aventura, FL**

"I have quite a few of your
Visual books and have been
very pleased with all of them.
I love the way the
lessons are presented!"

**Mary Jane Newman
Yorba Linda, CA**

"Like a lot of other people,
I understand things best
when I see them visually.
Your books really make
learning easy and
life more fun."

**John T. Frey
Cadillac, MI**

maranGraphics is a family-run business
located near Toronto, Canada.

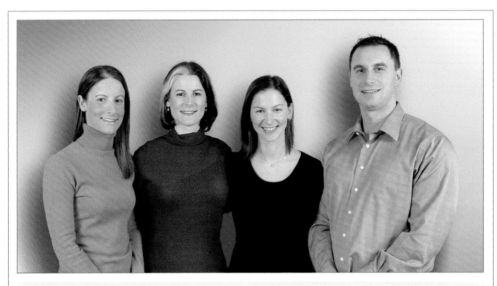

At **maranGraphics**, we believe in producing great consumer books– one book at a time.

Each maranGraphics book uses the award-winning communication process that we have been developing over the last 28 years. Using this process, we organize photographs and text in a way that makes it easy for you to learn new concepts and tasks.

We spend hours deciding the best way to perform each task, so you don't have to! Our clear, easy-to-follow photographs and instructions walk you through each task from beginning to end.

We want to thank you for purchasing what we feel are the best books money can buy. We hope you enjoy using this book as much as we enjoyed creating it!

Sincerely,

The Maran Family

Please visit us on the Web at:

www.maran.com

CREDITS

Author:
maranGraphics
Development Group

Content Architects:
Kelleigh Johnson
Wanda Lawrie

Technical Consultant:
Colleen Tiltman

Photography Consultant:
Anita Adler

Project Manager:
Judy Maran

Copy Development Director:
Jill Maran-Dutfield

Copy Development and Editing:
Roxanne Van Damme
Megan Robinson

Editing:
Raquel Scott
Roderick Anatalio

Layout Designer:
Sarah Jang

**Front Cover, Yoga Backgrounds
and Overviews:**
Designed by Russ Marini

Photographic Retouching:
Russ Marini
Steven Schaerer

Indexer:
Megan Robinson

**Wiley Vice President and
Executive Publisher:**
Kathy Nebenhaus

Wiley Staff:
Dawn Barnes
Roxane Cerda
Cindy Kitchel
Lisa Murphy
Susan Olinsky

Principal Model:
Elizabeth Clarke

Front Cover Model:
Jill Maran-Dutfield

Additional Models:
Anita Adler
Emma Bizi
Sandra Freedhoff
Richard Maran

**Photography and
Post Production:**
Robert Maran

ACKNOWLEDGMENTS

Thanks to the dedicated staff of maranGraphics, including Roderick Anatalio,
Sarah Jang, Kelleigh Johnson, Wanda Lawrie, Jill Maran, Judy Maran,
Robert Maran, Ruth Maran, Russ Marini, Megan Robinson,
Steven Schaerer, Raquel Scott and Roxanne Van Damme.

Finally, to Richard Maran who originated the easy-to-use graphic format
of this guide. Thank you for your inspiration and guidance.

ABOUT THE TECHNICAL CONSULTANT...

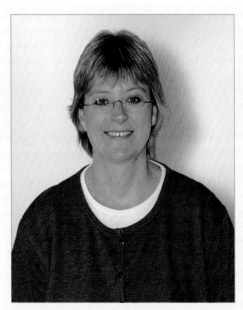

Colleen Tiltman, RYT

Colleen has been accredited with the highest level of study at the Yoga Alliance, achieving the 500-hour designation. The Yoga Alliance is one of the most established organizations for governing the national standards of yoga. Colleen is a practicing yoga teacher and certified yoga therapist. She received her yoga teacher certification through The International Sivananda Yoga Vedanta Center and has also completed the Professional Yoga Therapy program with Integrative Yoga Therapy (IYT). Colleen mentors students in the IYT Home Study program and Professional Yoga Therapy program. In addition to teaching yoga classes, Colleen has a private yoga therapy practice at The Lotus Center for Yoga and Health.

A few words from Colleen...

I would like to express my heartfelt thanks to my husband, Norm, for his continuing love, encouragement and support. Thank you to the maranGraphics writing team for their professional guidance, and special thanks to Kelleigh for her moral support throughout this project. I also wish to thank all of my teachers for leading the way and inspiring me to follow this path of yoga.

"Health is wealth. Peace of mind is happiness. Yoga shows the way."

-Swami Vishnu-Devananda

About the photography consultant...

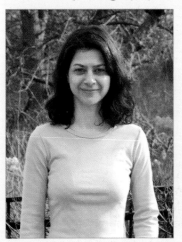

Anita Adler, RYT

Anita has been practicing yoga for over ten years. She received her teaching certificate from Esther Myers' Yoga Studio in the Vanda Scaravelli tradition of yoga. Anita is also certified in Pre and Post-Natal yoga. She is a Registered Yoga Alliance Teacher (500-hour).

Anita teaches ongoing classes in diverse settings such as the workplace, private homes, condominiums and community centers. She has taught seniors, children, athletes, pregnant women, mother and baby classes and yoga for people with multiple sclerosis. In addition to her classes, Anita offers workshops and retreats.

Anita holds degrees from York University in psychology and social work. She has worked with school boards, autistic children and troubled youth living in group homes.

About the model...

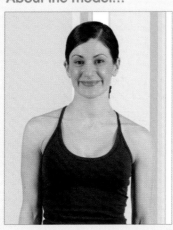

Elizabeth Clarke

Elizabeth fell in love with Yoga five years ago and hasn't looked back since. Today, she truly believes that the busier your life, the more you need yoga.

Balancing and flexibility used to mean juggling kids' schedules, full-time career and family life. Strength was developed by carrying heavy groceries. And then one fateful day, she accidentally found a yoga class at a community center. She grew to learn that practicing yoga completely spills over into your life in the most fantastic ways. It is truly a practice for the mind, body and spirit.

She is thankful to her wonderful children, Sam and Brianna for their ongoing inspiration to keep stretching herself. And to James, her fiancé, for proposing to a yogi.

Table of Contents

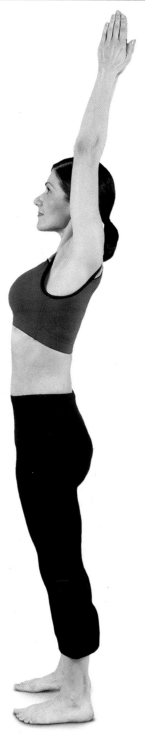

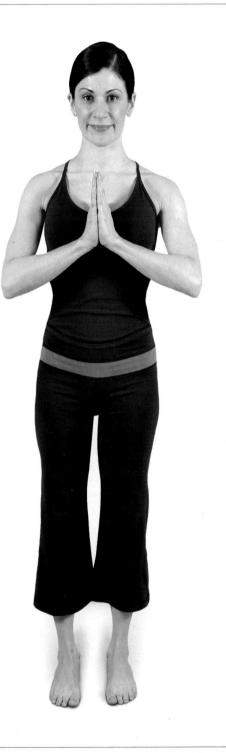

Table of Contents

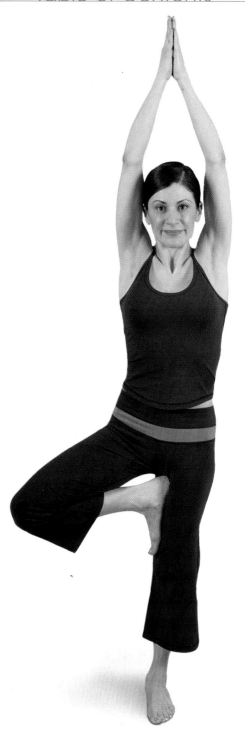

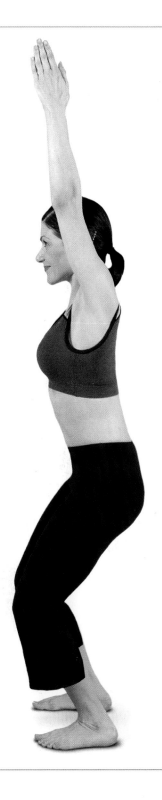

Table of Contents

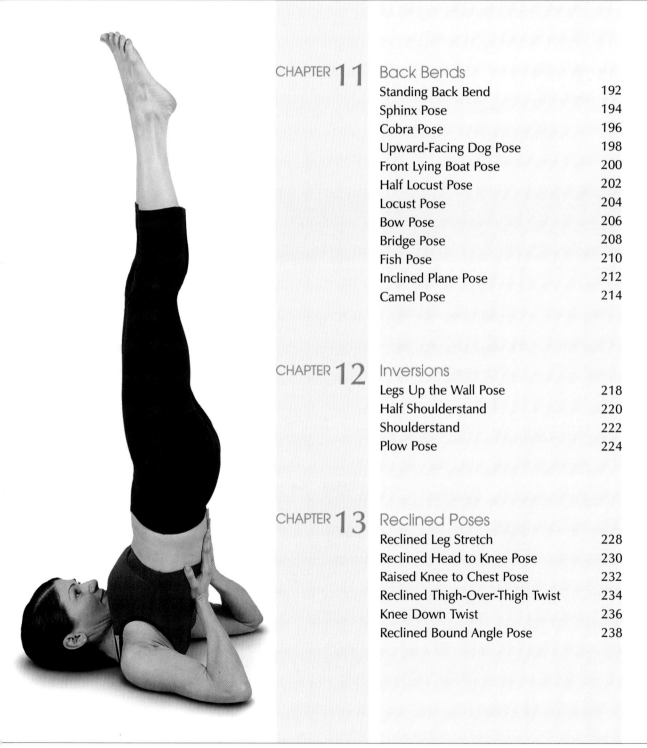

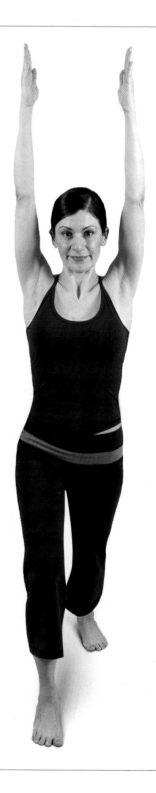

Chapter 1

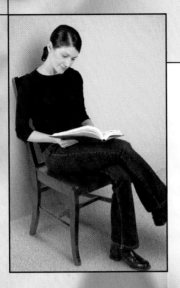

Yoga is beneficial for everyone, regardless of age or physical ability. The aim of practicing yoga is to improve your physical, mental and spiritual well-being. This chapter introduces you to the different types of yoga and explores the fundamentals of yoga, including relaxation, meditation and poses. You will also learn about the many benefits of yoga and how to incorporate this versatile activity into your lifestyle.

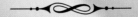

Yoga Basics

In this Chapter...

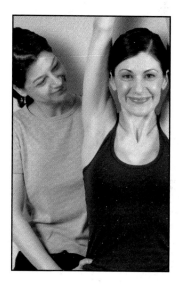

introduction to yoga

Although yoga has been around for thousands of years, it has recently gained widespread popularity throughout the world. Yoga is currently practiced by millions of people worldwide. Due to today's busy lifestyles, more and more people are discovering yoga as a means of relieving stress and improving their overall well-being.

What is Yoga?

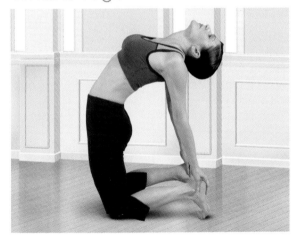

Yoga focuses on improving your physical, mental and spiritual well-being. The goal of yoga is to harmonize your body, mind and spirit through a combination of poses, meditation and breathing exercises. Unifying your body, mind and spirit allows you to achieve a sense of wholeness, peace and self-realization.

In addition to achieving inner peace, practicing yoga has many physical and mental benefits. For example, the physical exercise involved in yoga can increase your strength and flexibility. Yoga is also a very effective tool for relieving stress, calming your mind and allowing you to achieve complete physical and mental relaxation.

Who can practice Yoga?

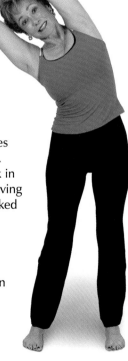
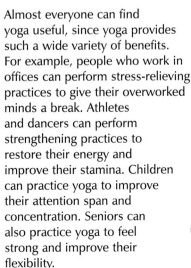

Anyone can practice yoga, regardless of age or fitness level. If you have a physical limitation, you can modify yoga to meet your needs. For instance, people with limited mobility can perform yoga while sitting in a chair.

Almost everyone can find yoga useful, since yoga provides such a wide variety of benefits. For example, people who work in offices can perform stress-relieving practices to give their overworked minds a break. Athletes and dancers can perform strengthening practices to restore their energy and improve their stamina. Children can practice yoga to improve their attention span and concentration. Seniors can also practice yoga to feel strong and improve their flexibility.

What does "Yoga" mean?

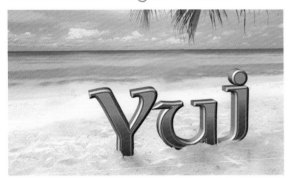

The word "yoga" is derived from the Sanskrit word "yuj," which means "to unify" or "to yoke."

This origin of the word "yoga" and the practice of yoga are closely related, since practicing yoga involves seeking to "unite" your body, mind and spirit. Achieving this union allows you to connect with your inner self, leading to a sense of contentment and tranquility.

How did Yoga begin?

Yoga originated in northern India more than 5,000 years ago. Archaeologists have found statuettes of men in yoga poses that are estimated to be 5,000 years old. Developed by the ancient sages of India, yoga was not written down for many thousands of years, but instead passed down from teacher to student. Approximately 2,000 years ago, a philosopher named Patanjali began to organize and write down the principles of yoga. Patanjali's collection of yoga's principles is known as *Yoga Sutras*. Many people consider Patanjali to be the father of yoga.

Why should I practice Yoga?

Yoga provides a balanced and wholesome approach to achieving good physical and mental health. To begin with, yoga is easier on your body than many other fitness activities, such as high-impact aerobics. Also, unlike many other forms of exercise, yoga addresses all aspects of your health and well-being. Breathing exercises can help you learn to breathe more efficiently. Meditation can clear your mind and help you stay calm. Yoga poses can provide many physical benefits, such as increasing your flexibility and improving your circulation.

Yoga also has mental and emotional benefits. For example, yoga can help improve your concentration, as well as soothe and rejuvenate your mind.

Yoga is increasingly being recognized for its value in preventing and relieving physical ailments, such as chronic back pain, arthritis and migraines.

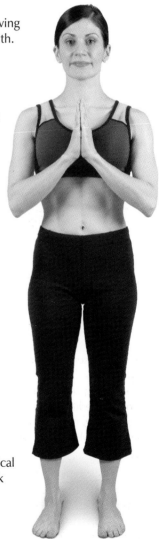

types of yoga

There are seven main types of yoga. Although each type of yoga helps unite your mind, body and spirit, each has a slightly different focus.

Hatha Yoga

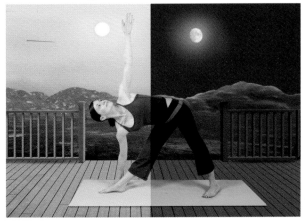

This book focuses on Hatha Yoga, which is the yoga of physical discipline. Hatha Yoga is the most commonly practiced type of yoga in the western world. The goal of Hatha Yoga is to achieve union of the mind, body and spirit through physical actions. Hatha Yoga promotes taking care of your body to be healthy.

The word *"Hatha"* is derived from two Sanskrit words—*"ha"* meaning *"sun"* and *"tha"* meaning *"moon."* The practice of Hatha Yoga finds a balance between your sun and moon traits and balances the opposites within you—from the right and left sides of your brain to the masculine and feminine sides of your personality.

The benefits of practicing Hatha Yoga may be felt immediately. Your body may become more relaxed and your mind may become clearer after just one practice. Some other benefits may occur with regular practice of Hatha Yoga, such as increased strength and proper posture.

Bhakti Yoga

Bhakti Yoga is the yoga of devotion and selfless love. Bhakti is derived from the Sanskrit word *"bhaj,"* which means "to serve." Practicing Bhakti Yoga involves devotion to a divine being, usually through practices such as singing, dancing, chanting and praying. Individuals who practice Bhakti Yoga also express this devotion and love in everyday life.

Karma Yoga

The main principle behind Karma Yoga is performing selfless service, without expecting to gain anything from the service. The service should be performed with honesty and integrity. An example of Karma Yoga is volunteering in your community to help others who are less fortunate.

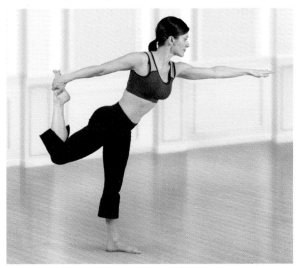

Jnana Yoga

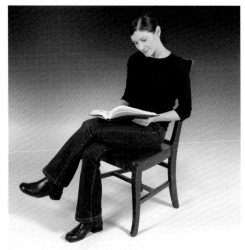

Jnana Yoga is the yoga of wisdom. In Sanskrit, the word *"Jnana"* means "knowledge," "insight," or "wisdom." One of the main principles of Jnana Yoga is to learn the distinction between what is real and unreal. Jnana Yoga also encourages humans to think of themselves as spiritual beings, who can reach enlightenment through willpower, study and reason.

Mantra Yoga

Mantra Yoga uses sound to heal your body and center and focus your mind. A mantra is a meditation technique in which you repeat a word aloud or silently in your mind. The most traditional mantra used is the word *"om."*

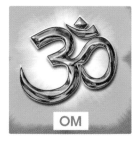

OM

Tantra Yoga

Tantra Yoga uses breath and movement to awaken the spiritual energy in your body. Two popular forms of Tantra Yoga are Kundalini Yoga and Kriya Yoga.

Raja Yoga

Raja Yoga, *"raja"* meaning "royal," is a classical type of yoga, in which meditation teaches your mind to serve your spirit.

The foundation of Raja Yoga is based on eight limbs. These limbs include:

1	Yama (Moral and Ethical Discipline)
2	Niyama (Self-discipline)
3	Asana (Poses)
4	Pranayama (Breath Control)
5	Pratyahara (Sensory Inhibition)
6	Dharana (Concentration)
7	Dhyana (Meditation)
8	Samadhi (Enlightenment)

what is hatha yoga?

The yoga poses included in this book are based on Hatha Yoga. The primary focus of Hatha Yoga is to unite your mind and body through the physical movement of poses, the awareness of your breath, and relaxation and meditation techniques. You can practice Hatha Yoga to increase your strength and flexibility, learn proper body alignment and improve your health and well-being.

TYPES OF HATHA YOGA

Ashtanga Yoga

Ashtanga Yoga, also called Power Yoga, is the most athletic type of Hatha Yoga. Developed by K. Pattabhi Jois, Ashtanga Yoga emphasizes intense stretching and building muscular strength. A specific series of poses and breathing exercises are practiced in order to heat up your body and sweat out toxins. The room temperature in which Ashtanga Yoga is practiced must be kept at approximately 70 to 75°F to keep your muscles supple.

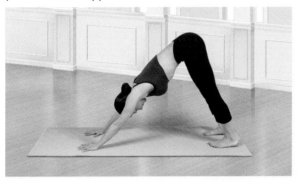

Bikram Yoga

Bikram Yoga is a popular type of yoga that was created by Bikram Choudhury. The Bikram Yoga practice consists of a sequence of 26 postures, which are each held for approximately 20 to 30 seconds. The room temperature in which Bikram Yoga is practiced should be approximately 105°F and 60% humidity. The heated room is beneficial for warming up your muscles to allow a deeper stretch and to detoxify your body.

Integral Yoga

Integral Yoga was originated by Swami Satchidananda. When practicing Integral Yoga, you participate in poses, breathing techniques, meditation and deep relaxation. Integral Yoga also emphasizes the importance of eating a healthy diet and service to humanity. Practitioners of Integral Yoga believe the purpose of a pose is more important than perfecting a pose.

Iyengar Yoga

Iyengar Yoga, established by B.K.S. Iyengar, makes extensive use of props, such as blocks, chairs and straps, to ensure the body is correctly aligned during a yoga pose. Iyengar Yoga also places emphasis on building strength and endurance, encouraging relaxation, increasing flexibility and relieving ailments.

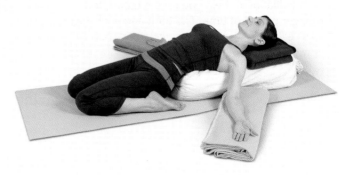

TYPES OF HATHA YOGA (CONTINUED)

Kundalini Yoga

Kundalini Yoga, sometimes referred to as the "mother yoga," was initiated by Yogi Bhajan. When practicing Kundalini Yoga, you practice poses, breathing, chanting and meditation to move energy through your body, specifically through your spine.

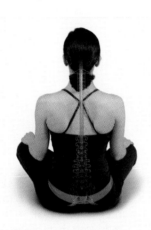

Kripalu Yoga

Kripalu Yoga was inspired by Kripalvananda. Kripalu is derived from the Sanskrit word "kripal," which means "compassion." This type of yoga emphasizes the importance of your mind and body being treated equally.

There are three stages to progress through when practicing Kripalu Yoga. In the first stage, you must focus on your alignment, breathing and movement, without concern for how long you can hold a pose. In the second stage, you can use meditation to help you hold the pose for a longer period of time. The third and final stage involves using meditation to allow your body to move instinctively from one position to another, depending on what feels right to you at the time.

Viniyoga

Viniyoga was developed by Shri Krishnamacharya and carried on by his son T.K.V. Desikachar. Krishnamacharya taught several well-known yoga gurus, including B.K.S. Iyengar. In Viniyoga, you practice poses that are gentle and relaxed. Instead of trying to achieve perfect form when you practice poses, you only need to practice to meet your needs and capabilities.

Sivananda Yoga

Swami Sivananda, who was a medical doctor, yoga master and world spiritual teacher, created Sivananda Yoga. This type of Hatha Yoga consists of a series of twelve poses: Headstand, Shoulderstand, Plow, Fish, Seated Forward Bend, Cobra, Locust, Bow, Spinal Twist, Crow, Standing Forward Bend and Triangle. Sivananda Yoga is based on five main principles: proper exercise, proper breathing, proper relaxation, proper diet and positive thinking and meditation.

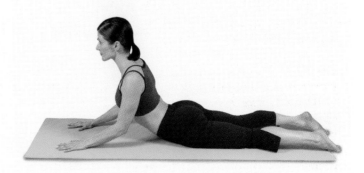

benefits of yoga

Yoga provides many benefits for men and women of all ages, from children to seniors.

Many yoga poses can be modified for people of all different levels of fitness and flexibility, even for people with temporary or chronic physical problems. The primary goal of yoga is to unite the mind, body and spirit. This union can improve your overall mental and physical well-being.

MENTAL AND EMOTIONAL BENEFITS

Improved Mood

Through the practice of yoga, you may find that you develop a more positive outlook on life. Practicing yoga encourages personal reflection and introspection, helping you to release any anxiety, hostility or depression you may be feeling. The peace and relaxation that yoga offers improves your mood, which in turn improves your overall well-being.

Stress Relief

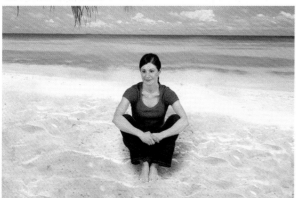

One of the most recognized benefits of yoga is stress reduction. The practice of yoga poses, meditation and breathing exercises are all clinically proven methods of relieving stress. Practicing yoga can help relieve stress by clearing your mind and bringing your attention to the present moment. Relieving stress can have a positive effect on your health, especially since medical practitioners consider stress to be the cause of many illnesses.

Improved Mental Functions

Yoga also serves as an effective tool to help improve your mental functioning. For example, you can enhance your memory and ability to concentrate through the practice of yoga. Many yoga poses can also improve your hand-eye coordination, reaction time, dexterity and fine motor skills.

Improved Self-Confidence

You can build greater self-confidence through the practice of yoga, especially because yoga is non-competitive. Yoga is an individual practice, which allows you to only focus on your own capabilities without comparing yourself to others. You can also improve your posture through the practice of yoga, which allows you to stand, sit and walk with confidence. Yoga can also make you feel more mentally alert, centered and content.

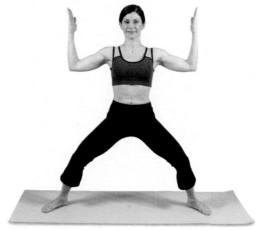

PHYSICAL BENEFITS

Pain Reduction

Yoga can provide therapeutic relief from many ailments, such as back pain, arthritis, migraine headaches and menstrual cramps. Many yoga poses can also release tension and soreness in your muscles. Practicing yoga can even help you prevent illness and injury by improving your immune system and teaching you to treat your body well. As a result, yoga can serve as preventative therapy to help you not only improve, but also maintain your health.

Improved Breathing

The practice of yoga improves your breathing by heightening your awareness of your breath and increasing your lung capacity. By focusing on deep breathing in your yoga practice, you can help to release tension from your body and make your body more alkaline and less acidic. Too much acidity in your body can be harmful for your bones and tissues, and can also cause arthritis, fatigue, headaches and depression.

Improved Circulation

Many yoga poses help to improve the circulation of blood throughout your body. Improved blood circulation helps flush out toxins and impurities from your body. Regular practice of yoga can also help lower your blood pressure and pulse rate.

Improved Strength and Flexibility

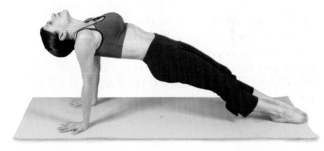

One of the most noticeable effects of yoga is that it can make your body strong and flexible, while improving the range of motion in your joints. The practice of yoga can also improve your balance, tone your muscles and increase your stamina. Some yoga poses can also help you build strong bones, which helps to prevent osteoporosis.

Additional Benefits

Yoga also provides a whole host of other health benefits. Through the practice of yoga, you can regulate your metabolism, which can help you lose weight. Yoga also helps to balance your hormonal system, which is especially useful for menopausal and pre-menopausal women. In addition, the movement in some yoga poses massages the internal organs of the body, which improves certain bodily functions, such as digestion and elimination.

yoga clothes and props

YOGA CLOTHES

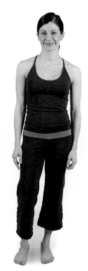

You should wear clothes that are comfortable and allow you to move and breathe freely when practicing yoga. Wearing flexible clothing is the best option, such as a leotard, leggings or bicycle shorts, because your clothing will not move or get in your way. You can also wear a T-shirt and gym shorts if you feel more comfortable. You may want to layer your clothing so you can take layers off as you warm up and put layers back on as you cool down.

Yoga is best practiced barefoot. When you are barefoot, you are better able to feel the floor beneath your feet. Wearing socks may cause you to slip.

YOGA PROPS

Yoga Mat

A yoga mat, also called a sticky mat, is a thin, rectangular rubber mat that helps keep you from sliding on the floor as you move into various poses. A yoga mat is also made of material that is the appropriate texture. If you practice on a surface that is too soft, such as carpet, you may find it difficult to balance or position yourself correctly. If you try to practice on a hard surface, such as hardwood, some poses may be too uncomfortable for your hands, knees or feet.

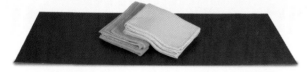

Blankets

Keep a few large wool or cotton blankets nearby when practicing yoga. A folded blanket can protect your knees when kneeling. You can also use folded blankets to provide support for your body, such as placing a blanket under your head in a lying pose.

Yoga Strap

A yoga strap is a long cotton band, which may or may not have a buckle, and is usually $1\frac{1}{2}$ inches wide and 6 feet long. The yoga strap is a useful aid when you cannot reach a part of your body with your hands. If you do not have a yoga strap, you can use any soft cloth or belt, such as a bathrobe belt.

Chair

You may need to use a sturdy chair with a back and a flat seat when performing some standing poses or seated chair poses. You should use an armless chair for seated chair poses.

YOGA PROPS (CONTINUED)

Wall

You can use a wall to help you maintain correct posture, alignment or balance in a yoga pose. Walls are particularly helpful for poses such as standing balancing poses.

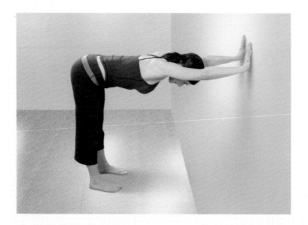

Bolsters

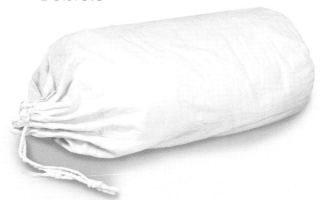

Bolsters are cylindrical or rectangular pillows that measure approximately 8 inches high and 26 inches long. They are usually covered with canvas or cotton and stuffed with cotton batting to make them firm. Bolsters are useful if you need a firm surface to prop up or rest your body on. If you do not have a bolster, you can roll up a blanket, stack folded blankets or use a firm sofa or bed pillow.

Blocks

Blocks are usually 4 x 6 x 9 inches in size and made of either foam or wood. For your yoga practice, you will most likely find two blocks useful. If you do not have a block, you can create your own block by wrapping a hardcover book with tape.

Blocks are helpful when your hands cannot reach down to the floor, such as in a standing twist. You can place any end of the block on the floor to achieve the height you need, but make sure the block is steady. Do not clutch the block, but only rest your hand on it to keep your balance.

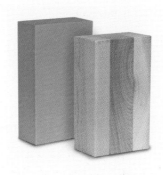

Eye Bag

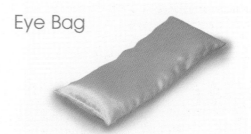

An eye bag is a small cloth bag usually filled with flax seeds. Covering your eyes with an eye bag during a relaxation pose helps relax your eyes and face and block the light. If you do not have an eye bag, use a folded washcloth or silk scarf as a substitute.

creating a
yoga environment

If you would like to practice yoga on your own, you can create a yoga environment in your home. Once you create a yoga environment, you can begin practicing yoga with the aid of books, videos and audio recordings. You may want to practice yoga with a qualified yoga teacher to ensure that you understand the basics before practicing on your own.

What time of day should I practice yoga?

You can practice yoga at any time in the day when you feel you need to. Performing an active yoga practice in the morning can energize your mind and body, which can help set the tone for how you feel the rest of the day. You may want to perform a less active practice in the evening to help calm your mind and body after a long day and prepare yourself for sleep. Try to set a specific time each day, or as often in the week as possible, to practice yoga so your practice will become a habit.

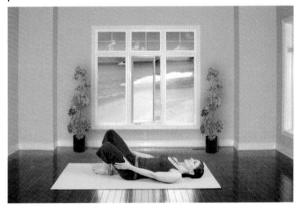

Where should I practice?

When practicing at home, you should create an area specifically for yoga and meditation. Make sure there is plenty of sunlight and that the area is clean and tidy. Also, make sure you do not have any distractions while you practice yoga.

Should I be concerned about the air quality?

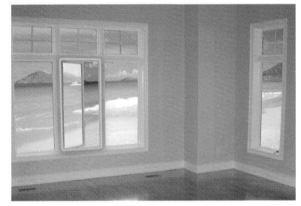

Yes. If possible, you should open a window to allow fresh air to come in. Fresh air is especially beneficial for your breathing, which is integral to yoga. Also, make sure the air is not polluted with burning incense, smoke or any other type of air pollution.

How else should I prepare my yoga environment?

Make sure every prop you need for your practice, such as a yoga mat, blankets and blocks, are in the area before you begin. This preparation prevents you from having to run around the house looking for a different prop before you perform each pose.

finding a
yoga class

You should consider joining a yoga class, especially if you are a beginner. You may want to take at least a few classes with a qualified yoga teacher before practicing completely on your own. A yoga teacher can work with you to make sure you are doing poses correctly and safely. If you are a beginner, make sure you sign up for a beginner yoga class.

Questions to Ask Yourself

Do I want to take a group class or take private lessons?

Do I want the class to take place at a yoga center, yoga studio, fitness club or private home?

How much time do I have to devote to going to a yoga class?

How much money do I want to spend on a yoga class?

Where to Find a Yoga Class

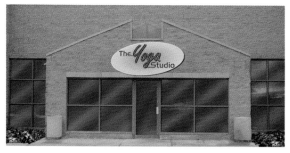

Word of mouth is the most common way to find a yoga class. You can also look in the Yellow Pages, online resources and in natural food stores for business cards or flyers. Your local community center or fitness club may also offer yoga classes.

Many courses are offered in sessions, often in the fall, winter and spring. Some locations offer drop-in classes, which are useful if you want to try a class without having to sign up for an entire session.

Questions to Ask a Yoga Teacher

What yoga training do you have?
Yoga teachers can be certified by certain schools of yoga where the training can vary from one week to a few years.

What yoga experience do you have?
Although a teacher may not be certified, he or she may have many valuable years of teaching experience.

Are you able to accommodate any physical limitations that I have?
If your problems are serious, you should consult your doctor before practicing yoga.

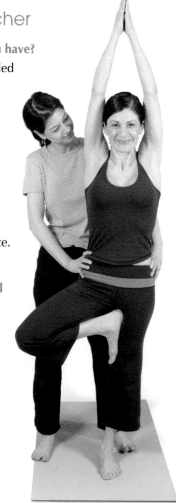

yoga and relaxation

Yoga attracts many people as a means of relaxation. Common methods of relaxing, such as watching television or chatting with friends, serve more as a distraction than a means of achieving complete relaxation. Yoga teaches your body and mind to relax completely by consciously releasing both physical and mental tension. You can achieve this relaxation through the practice of yoga poses, breath awareness and relaxation techniques. In fact, relaxation is so important in yoga that a portion of every practice should be entirely devoted to relaxation.

TYPES OF RELAXATION

Physical Relaxation

Yoga poses are extremely beneficial for relaxing your body. As you stretch and move your body in a yoga practice, you can release tension from your muscles, allowing them to relax. Yoga allows you to connect with your body and become aware of any tension that may be present. Through your yoga practice, you can focus on relaxing any areas that may require attention.

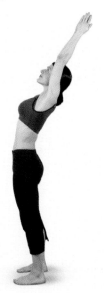

Mental Relaxation

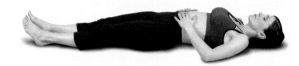

Yoga provides you with an opportunity to set aside time each day to allow your mind to relax and unwind. By taking time each day to practice yoga, you can help prevent your mind from becoming overwhelmed and fatigued. The practice of breath awareness is especially useful for relaxing your mind. For more information on breath awareness, see pages 34 to 39.

Spiritual Relaxation

Once you achieve physical and mental relaxation, spiritual relaxation is also possible. Spiritual relaxation brings a feeling of inner peace and contentment. This type of relaxation also promotes a sense of inner awareness, which can help put you in touch with yourself and those around you.

BENEFITS OF RELAXATION

Relaxation is necessary for your mental and physical well-being. If you do not give yourself time to relax on a regular basis, your body and mind can become worn out and overwhelmed. Relaxation is the most natural and effective way to soothe and revitalize your mind. Through relaxation, you will become more in touch with your body, enabling you to recognize and overcome any tension in your body more easily.

RELAXATION TECHNIQUES

Guided Imagery and Guided Relaxation

Guided imagery and guided relaxation are relaxation techniques in which you listen to a message specifically designed for relaxation. You can work with a partner or use a recording of your own voice or another voice reading a relaxation script. You can also purchase guided imagery and guided relaxation audio recordings.

To prepare for guided imagery or guided relaxation, you should make sure your environment is quiet and free from distractions. Begin in Relaxation Pose, as shown on page 242, and place an eye bag or folded face cloth over your eyes. During guided imagery or guided relaxation, your mind and body work together to help you achieve a state of deep relaxation.

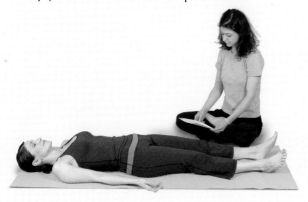

Yoga Nidra

Yoga Nidra is a powerful relaxation technique where you remain aware and conscious as you move into a state of deep relaxation. This state of complete mental and physical relaxation heals and rejuvenates your entire body and mind. You should work with an experienced yoga instructor to explore the Yoga Nidra technique.

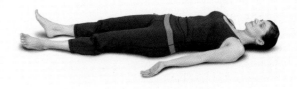

Tense-Relax Technique

The Tense-Relax Technique involves moving through your entire body, tensing each part of your body and then releasing the part and allowing it to completely relax.

To perform Tense-Relax Technique, begin in Relaxation Pose. Inhale and tense your feet, hold for a moment and then exhale and release your feet, allowing the tension to drain away. Inhale slowly and then exhale slowly, allowing your feet to completely relax. Continue to tense and release each part of your body, gradually moving up to your head.

yoga and meditation

Meditation is an important aspect of yoga that can strengthen the union of your mind, body and spirit. Meditation provides you with an opportunity to sit still, clear your mind of all thoughts and fully relax your body.

The practice of meditation may also help you develop a sense of spiritual strength and peacefulness. Although meditation involves a spiritual element, yoga is not a religion.

You should meditate every day, starting with 5 minute sessions and working up to 20 or 30 minutes.

MEDITATION TECHNIQUES

Preparing for Meditation

To help you stay focused as you meditate, you should create an environment that is quiet and free from distractions. Also, try to practice at the same time every day, which can help you make your meditation practice a habit.

The position in which you sit is also important for helping you stay focused during your meditation practice. Sit cross-legged, always making sure your spine is upright and straight. You can either sit on the floor, on a straight-backed chair or on a meditation cushion. A meditation cushion is a pillow that is designed to help you sit straight and comfortably as you meditate.

You can meditate with your eyes closed or open, whichever you find helps you stay focused. Just make sure that your eyes remain relaxed at all times.

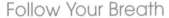

Follow Your Breath

Focusing on your breath can help you meditate. If you find your mind wanders while meditating, try to bring your attention back to your breath. It may also be helpful to use techniques that remind you to follow your breath. For example, you can mentally say "inhale" on each inhalation and "exhale" on each exhalation. You could also count your breaths by mentally saying "inhale one, exhale two…" and so on.

Use a Mantra

A mantra is a meditation technique in which you repeat a word, such as "love," "peace," or *"om"* as you meditate. You can either repeat the word aloud or silently in your mind.

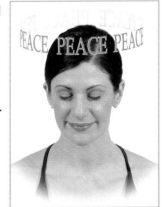

yoga and your lifestyle

Yoga is suitable for people of all ages and abilities. If you choose to adopt yoga as part of your lifestyle, you can improve your physical, mental and spiritual well-being. Incorporating yoga into your daily life does not simply involve practicing yoga poses. Yoga may also influence other aspects of your lifestyle, such as your outlook on life, your relationships with others and your health and diet.

Attitude

Practicing yoga helps you develop a positive attitude toward yourself and others. Yoga also encourages positive human traits, such as understanding, patience and love. You can also develop an increased sense of awareness, which can make you more alert and responsive to your surroundings. You should strive to bring this positive attitude, awareness and sense of peace into your daily life.

Yoga Practice

A complete yoga practice includes meditation, poses and relaxation. By practicing yoga, you will become stronger, healthier and experience increased energy that can positively affect many other areas of your life. To benefit most from your practice, try to make your yoga practice a daily habit by practicing at the same time and place each day.

Healthy Diet

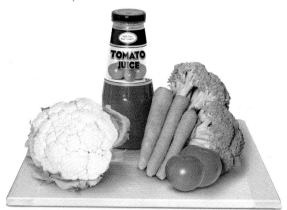

An important part of a complete yoga practice is healthy eating. When shopping for groceries, you should select food that is natural, nutritious and unprocessed. Good choices include fresh fruits and vegetables, grains, nuts, whole grain breads and dairy products.

You should avoid foods that may overstimulate your mind and body, such as refined sugar, caffeine and alcohol. Also, try to avoid foods that can make you feel sluggish, such as meat, fried foods and fast food.

yoga and pregnancy

Yoga can be very beneficial and therapeutic for pregnant women. Practicing yoga not only helps physically prepare a woman for childbirth, but it can also positively influence her mental and emotional state to prepare her for this life-changing experience.

It is best to start practicing yoga before you become pregnant. This allows you to become more familiar with yoga and allows your body to adjust to your yoga practice before the onset of the changes that come with the early stages of pregnancy.

If you are pregnant, it is important that you discuss practicing yoga with your doctor before you begin, regardless of whether you have practiced yoga before. You should then try to find a prenatal yoga class taught by a qualified teacher.

Physical Benefits

Yoga can ease many physical problems involved in pregnancy. For example, performing yoga poses can help relieve fatigue, nausea, heartburn, leg cramps and varicose veins. Practicing yoga also helps you maintain good posture throughout your pregnancy, which can help alleviate backache. Through practicing yoga, you can learn breathing and relaxation techniques that you can use during labor to help you cope with any pain you experience.

Mental and Emotional Benefits

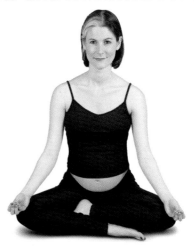

Yoga can help you deal with any mental and emotional stress you may experience during pregnancy and childbirth. Yoga can teach you to focus and concentrate, which can help you through the course of your pregnancy as well as during labor.

Yoga can also help you deal with mood swings, as well as anxiety and fear about childbirth. By heightening your awareness of your body, yoga can increase the confidence you have in your body's ability to give birth. You may also find that you can discover a deeper connection with your unborn baby through meditation.

CAUTIONS DURING PREGNANCY

Avoid Poses on Your Back

After the first trimester of your pregnancy, you should avoid poses that require you to lie flat on your back for a long period of time. When you lie on your back, the weight of the fetus can restrict the flow of blood in your lower body.

Avoid Putting Pressure on Your Abdomen

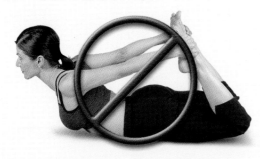

When you are pregnant, you should avoid poses that require you to lie on your belly or other poses that put pressure on your abdomen, such as forward bends and twists. However, you can modify forward bends and twists to make them safe for pregnancy. You should seek advice from a qualified yoga teacher to learn how to modify poses during your pregnancy.

Listen to Your Body

If you feel any discomfort or strain while performing a pose, you should come out of the pose immediately. You should also move slowly between poses. You will probably need to modify most poses when you are pregnant to accommodate the changes your body is going through.

Avoid Over-Stretching Your Muscles

During pregnancy, try not to stretch as far as you normally would. You should avoid poses that involve intense stretches, especially poses that stretch your abdominal muscles. There is also an increased danger of straining your muscles when you are pregnant because pregnancy hormones loosen the connective tissues in your body.

Avoid Inverted Poses and Back Bends

During pregnancy, you should avoid inverted poses, such as Shoulderstand. However, you can lie on the floor with the soles of your feet against a wall or your calves resting on a chair, provided you are not lying on your back for an extended period of time.

You should also avoid back bends during pregnancy. Because of the extra weight you carry on the front of your body when you are pregnant, these poses put additional pressure on your spine and lower back and can lead to back injury.

yoga for children

Yoga can be a great source of exercise, relaxation and fun for children. In fact, yoga is taught in many elementary schools in the United States. Yoga is especially beneficial for hyperactive children or children with Attention Deficit Disorder.

Finding a yoga class in your area that is designed for children may be difficult, but you should be able to find many books and videos about yoga for children. Remember that a yoga practice can only hold a child's attention for a limited amount of time. Aim for a 15 to 20 minute practice for children in preschool, a 20 to 30 minute practice for elementary school children and 30 minutes or more for preteens. Try to include at least a short period of relaxation at the end of each practice.

Making Yoga Fun

Always remember to make yoga fun for children. Try to turn yoga into a game that your child will enjoy. For example, have your child watch an animal, such as a cat, dog, frog, bear or lion, and then encourage him or her to imitate the animal's movements. There are many yoga poses that are based on imitating animals, such as Cat Stretch, Downward-Facing Dog Pose, Lion Pose and Cobra Pose. You can add a playful element to these poses by meowing, barking, roaring and hissing.

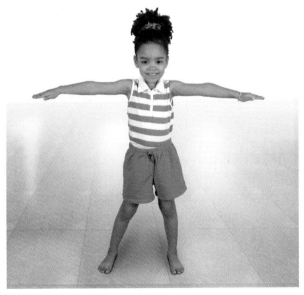

Benefits of Yoga for Children

PHYSICAL BENEFITS

Practicing yoga can help a child develop a greater awareness of his or her body and what it can do. Yoga can also increase strength and flexibility, improve balance and coordination and enhance a child's overall health.

MENTAL AND EMOTIONAL BENEFITS

Yoga is a great tool for stimulating children's imagination and creativity. Children can also become more confident and self-aware by practicing yoga. Yoga also teaches children how to focus and concentrate, which can improve their attention span. Moreover, yoga can help relieve stress in children and help them to better manage negative feelings and anger.

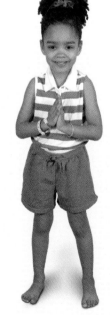

yoga for seniors

Yoga can be modified to suit the needs of seniors. Practicing yoga can help ease many of the physical problems experienced by seniors. In fact, yoga is becoming increasingly recognized as a good alternative to prescription drugs and invasive medical procedures. If you are a senior citizen, make sure you discuss practicing yoga with your doctor before you begin.

Why do seniors need yoga?

Seniors may not be very active and may also suffer from poor posture. These conditions can lead to weak muscles, back pain, joint stiffness, obesity, constipation, insomnia and depression. Also, seniors may experience problems with circulation, which can contribute to reduced mobility and general health problems.

What makes yoga a good choice for seniors?

Yoga is a gentle, easy and natural method of improving overall health and quality of life for all people, regardless of age or physical condition. Many yoga poses can be modified so they can be performed in a chair (as shown on pages 110 to 117), a wheelchair or even in bed.

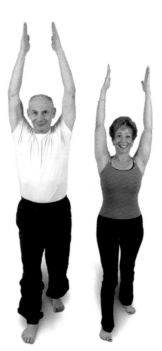

What are the benefits of yoga for seniors?

PHYSICAL BENEFITS

Yoga involves safe and gentle movements that effectively tone and strengthen muscles, increase flexibility and restore vitality. These benefits provide greater control over the body, which can help improve seniors' ability to move around safely. Yoga can also improve breathing, encourage relaxation and help people better cope with discomfort or pain. In addition, practicing yoga can help alleviate specific physical conditions suffered by many seniors, such as the symptoms of arthritis.

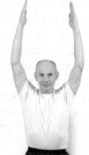

MENTAL AND EMOTIONAL BENEFITS

Participating in yoga classes provides social interaction, which encourages seniors to make new friends and feel a sense of community. The overall feeling of well-being that yoga offers can also lead to a positive attitude toward life. Yoga can provide the calm and serenity needed to alleviate depression and anxiety. Moreover, as people's flexibility, strength and energy increase, their confidence will grow.

muscular system

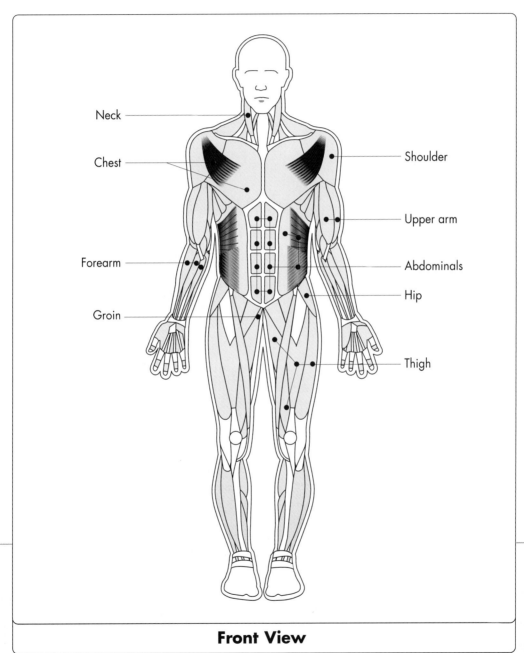

Neck

Chest

Forearm

Groin

Shoulder

Upper arm

Abdominals

Hip

Thigh

Front View

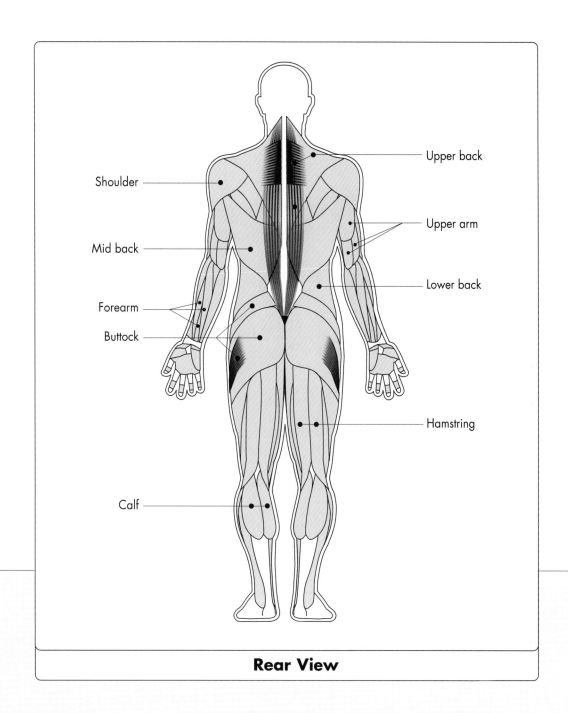

Upper back

Shoulder

Upper arm

Mid back

Lower back

Forearm

Buttock

Hamstring

Calf

Rear View

skeletal system

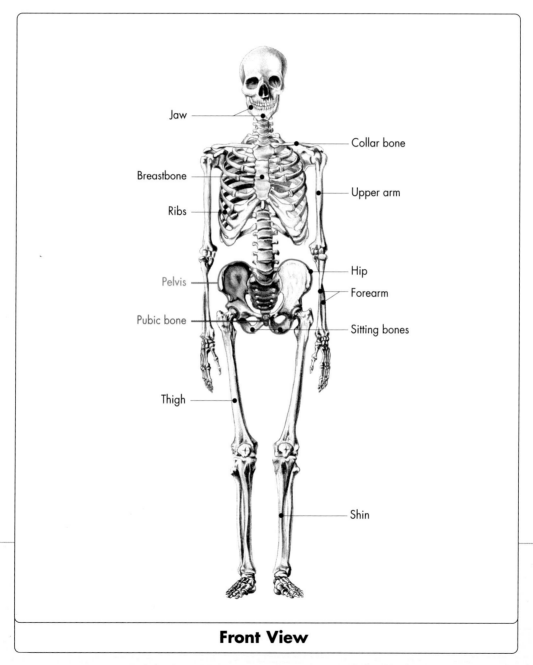

Jaw

Collar bone

Breastbone

Upper arm

Ribs

Pelvis

Hip

Forearm

Pubic bone

Sitting bones

Thigh

Shin

Front View

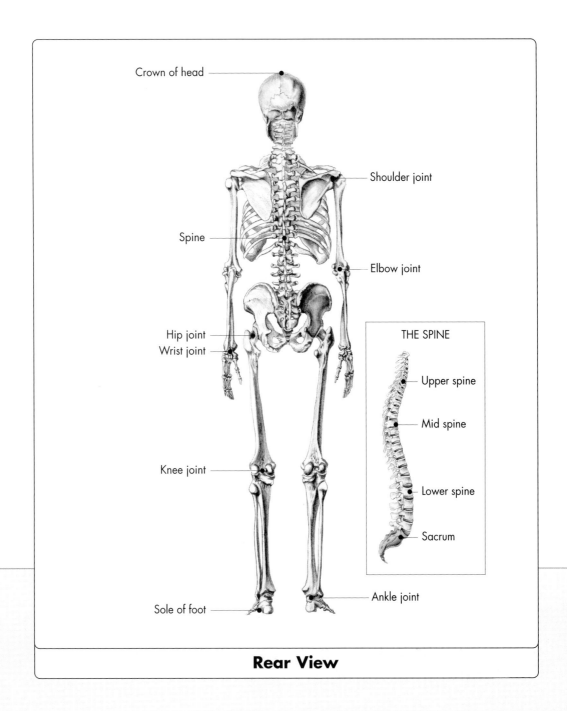

Crown of head

Shoulder joint

Spine

Elbow joint

Hip joint

Wrist joint

THE SPINE

Upper spine

Mid spine

Lower spine

Sacrum

Knee joint

Ankle joint

Sole of foot

Rear View

introduction to poses

This book includes over 90 yoga poses you can try at home. In Sanskrit, the word "pose" is *"asana"* (pronounced ah-sah-nah). Each *asana* helps you become more aware of your body, mind and environment. As you begin your yoga practice, allow yourself to experiment with the poses, moving into or out of the poses as you feel comfortable. Also, try to approach the poses with playful curiosity and without frustration or competitiveness. You should also never feel pain or discomfort when practicing a pose.

BREATHING AND POSES

Breathing is an essential part of practicing yoga poses. You should never hold your breath during a pose. Also, make sure your breath never feels forced or strained. Labored breathing is a strong indication that you are working too hard and should come out of the pose slightly.

Each pose described in this book

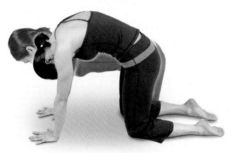

provides a guideline for how long to hold the pose. It is not necessary to follow this guideline exactly. When you begin practicing yoga, you can hold most poses for three full breaths and then evaluate how your body feels. If you feel comfortable in the pose, hold the pose for longer. If you feel uncomfortable, you should come out of the pose.

TYPES OF POSES

Seated Poses

Seated poses are useful for practicing breathing exercises and relaxation or meditation techniques. Seated poses are also often used as a warm up or as a starting point for other poses. Performing seated poses can help improve your posture and open your hips.

Standing Poses

Standing poses are often used as a warm-up or as a starting point for other poses. Standing poses are beneficial for strengthening your legs, opening your hips and improving your sense of balance.

Inversions

Inversions are excellent poses to perform to improve your blood circulation, quiet your mind and improve your overall health. Inversions are also believed to reverse the aging process and reduce the effect of gravity on your body.

TYPES OF POSES (CONTINUED)

Relaxation and Restorative Poses

It is important to take time to perform relaxation or restorative poses at the end of each yoga practice. You can use this time to relax your body and mind and allow energy released by the poses in your practice to move freely throughout your body.

Counter Poses

A counter pose is a pose that stretches your spine in the opposite direction from a previous pose or returns your spine to a neutral position. For example, after performing a back bend, such as Cobra Pose, you may want to perform a forward bend, such as Child's Pose, as a counter pose.

Twists

You can perform twists to stretch and strengthen your back and abdominal muscles, increase the flexibility of your spine and improve your circulation. Twists improve the functioning of your internal organs by providing them with a fresh supply of blood as you twist and release your body.

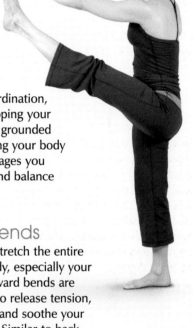

Balancing Poses

Balancing poses are great for improving your balance and coordination, as well as developing your ability to remain grounded in a pose. Keeping your body balanced encourages you to focus, quiet and balance your mind.

Forward Bends

Forward bends stretch the entire back of your body, especially your hamstrings. Forward bends are also often used to release tension, calm your mind and soothe your nervous system. Similar to back bends, forward bends help keep your spine strong and supple.

Back Bends

Back bends are among the most challenging poses in yoga. Bending backward helps strengthen your back and keep your spine strong and supple. Back bends also open the front of your body, especially your chest.

tips for a great
yoga practice

How should I approach my yoga practice?

You should approach your yoga practice with a positive attitude. When you first start practicing, you should set goals that are within your reach and try not to push yourself too hard. Yoga is about doing your best and learning how to accept yourself for who you are.

You may want to keep a yoga journal to record your growth as you practice yoga. You can include items in your yoga journal such as your thoughts, feelings and physical progress.

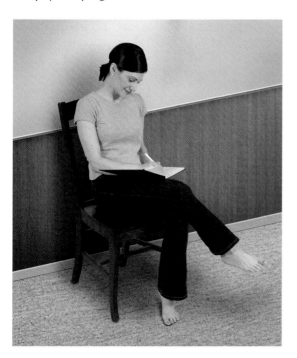

When should I practice?

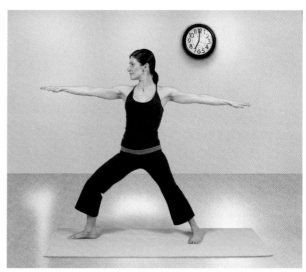

You should practice yoga at a time that is most convenient for you. This can help make your practice a daily habit. It is better to practice for a short time each day than to practice for a longer time less frequently. Although yoga practices normally last from 45 to 90 minutes, you may find there are days when you do not have enough time to fit in a full practice. In this case, you should at least take a few minutes to practice. Even a few minutes of yoga can have lasting benefits.

Should I eat before I practice?

It is best to practice yoga on an empty stomach, such as before breakfast or dinner. If you have eaten recently, consider waiting 2 to 3 hours before you practice. The length of time you should wait depends on what you have eaten. The heavier the meal, the longer you should wait before practicing. You should also avoid smoking or drinking alcohol or caffeine before a yoga practice.

THE POSES

Make Your Practice Enjoyable

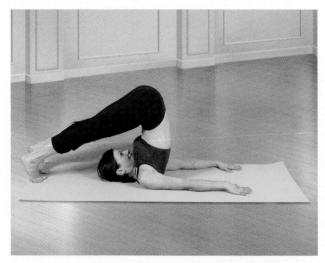

You will be more likely to continue practicing yoga if you make the experience enjoyable. Try to remain positive about the poses, rather than making it a competition to see how well you can perform each pose. You can also add variety to your routine by performing different poses every day. When you begin your practice, start with the poses you enjoy and that you feel offer the greatest benefit. You may want to try three or four poses to begin and then adjust your practice to suit your needs.

Balance Your Practice

You should make sure your practice is balanced. A balanced practice includes all three movements of the spine: forward bends, back bends and twists. It is also important to include shoulder and hip movements in your practice.

Listen to Your Body

Make sure you take a few moments to breathe and center yourself before you begin your practice. When practicing yoga, you should always listen to your body. Never push yourself into a pose that causes you to feel pain or discomfort. Instead, move slowly in and out of the poses so that you feel comfortable at all times. Consider each pose as a journey that consists of three parts: coming into the pose, holding the pose and coming out of the pose. All three parts of the pose are equally important.

You should always end your practice with a relaxation or restorative pose, such as Relaxation Pose. This relaxation time will help you fully integrate and absorb the benefits of your yoga practice.

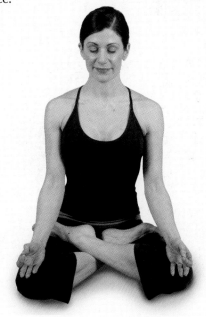

Chapter 2

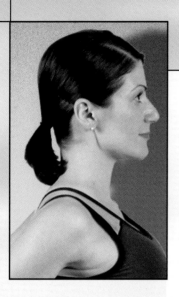

Breathing efficiently can positively influence your physical and mental well-being. For this reason, proper breathing is integral to the practice of yoga. This chapter shows you how to breathe efficiently to boost your energy and help rid your body of toxins. You will also learn how proper breathing techniques can clear your mind, improve your concentration and reduce stress. Perform the exercises in this chapter to help improve your breathing.

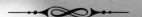

Yoga and Breathing

In this Chapter...

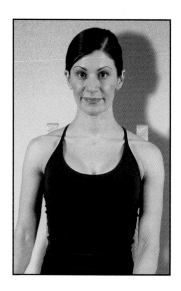

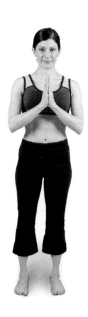

introduction to breathing

Although breathing is an involuntary bodily function, you can learn to control your breathing to adjust how your body responds to external circumstances.

Your breath connects your mind and your body, so becoming more aware of your breath can positively affect you both physically and mentally. When you bring awareness to your breathing, you also give yourself time to turn your attention inward and focus on your thoughts and emotions.

How do I know if I am breathing efficiently?

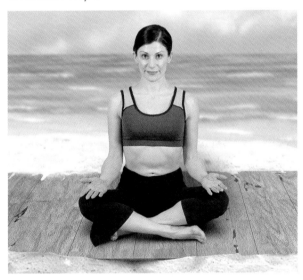

To ensure you are breathing efficiently, make sure your posture is correct, your spine is straight and your shoulders are relaxed. Proper posture helps ensure your lungs have the maximum amount of room to expand in your chest, which allows you to take full breaths. Taking full breaths maximizes the energy you bring into your body. You will also know if you are breathing efficiently when your breath is smooth and even. You may also feel your jaw relax, your shoulders drop away from your ears and your head and neck muscles relax.

Physical Benefits of Efficient Breathing

Breathing efficiently can relieve many ailments, including fatigue, sleep disorders, anxiety, dizziness, visual problems and chest problems. You can also keep your lung tissue elastic, tone your abdominal muscles and strengthen your immune system. As you breathe deeply, you increase your oxygen intake which boosts your energy, improves your metabolism and helps rid your body of toxins.

Mental Benefits of Efficient Breathing

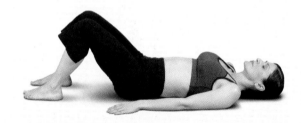

Breathing efficiently is not only beneficial for your body, but can also clear your mind, improve your concentration and reduce stress.

If you are upset or anxious, your breath may become quick and shallow. Through breathing exercises, you can control your breathing, which will restore a sense of calm.

YOGA AND BREATHING

Yoga, particularly Hatha Yoga, requires you to be constantly aware of your breath. As you breathe in your yoga practice, you exercise your diaphragm, abdominal muscles, heart, lungs and the muscles

that connect your ribs. It is best to breathe through your nose to filter the air your body takes in. You should try to take at least a few minutes each day for breath awareness.

Prana

Prana is the life force and energy that sustains all living things. As you breathe, prana flows throughout the cells in your body, making you strong and healthy. The goal of breathing efficiently is to balance the prana in your body and open areas that may be blocked. Visualizing this flow of energy helps to focus your mind and improve your awareness of the flow of prana in your body.

Tips for Better Breathing

The best place to perform breathing exercises is in a location with lots of fresh, clean, warm air. Make sure you do not wear any clothing that constricts your breathing, such as pants with a tight waistline. If you have lung problems, such as asthma, or if you have heart disease, you should consult your doctor before you perform breathing exercises.

Breathing During Poses

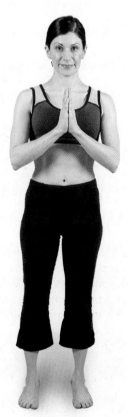

Your breath is an important element of performing any yoga pose. Focusing on your breathing may sharpen your concentration, prevent injury and help you release further into a pose. If your breathing becomes strained or forced, it may be an indication that you are working too hard.

When performing a yoga pose, make sure you never hold your breath. You should try to breathe evenly and deeply throughout the pose. In addition, you should try to match your breathing to the way you are moving in a pose. For example, you will usually inhale when you lift your arms, lengthen your body or bend backward. You will usually exhale when lowering your arms, bending forward or deepening a twist.

breath awareness exercise

This breath awareness exercise helps you connect with the natural rhythm of your breath and thereby increase your awareness of your breath. Practicing this breath awareness exercise before you begin your yoga practice helps center your mind and prepare you for the practice.

As you exhale, try to release the tension from your body. As you release your body's tension and begin to relax, your breath will become slower and more even. As you inhale, your breath should effortlessly fill your body. Your breath should gradually deepen as you perform this exercise.

While performing this exercise, do not try to regulate your breath or force yourself to breathe in a certain way. The purpose of the exercise is to discover and explore your breath, so you should simply notice how you breathe naturally. Once you have gained a greater awareness of your breath, you will be able to learn to control how you breathe.

You can practice this exercise lying down or while in a comfortable seated pose, such as Easy Pose.

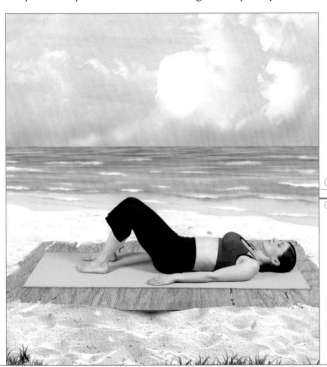 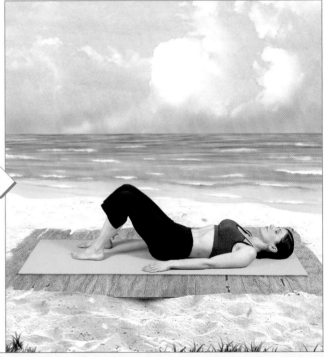

1 Lie on your back with your knees bent and the soles of your feet on the floor, hip width apart.

2 Inhale through your nose.

- Notice which parts of your body move and expand as you inhale.
- Feel your breath creating space and openness within your body.

3 Exhale through your nose.

- Listen to your breath.

- Notice which parts of your body move and release as you exhale.

4 Repeat steps 2 and 3 for 2 to 5 minutes.

abdominal breath

This abdominal breath exercise improves your ability to breathe more fully and deeply by increasing the air flow to the lower part of your lungs. You may also find that this exercise helps to calm and relax your body and mind.

As you perform this exercise, you should become aware of the rise and fall of your breath in your abdomen. As you breathe, make sure you do not tighten your abdominal muscles or press your abdomen outward. Your abdomen should expand naturally and remain soft throughout the exercise.

You can perform this exercise while lying in Relaxation Pose or sitting in a comfortable seated pose, such as Easy Pose. You can also perform this exercise while sitting in a chair, which is useful if you spend your day sitting at a desk. If you need more support for your lower back in Relaxation Pose, you can bend your knees and place the soles of your feet on the floor hip width apart.

You should be careful performing this exercise if you have low blood pressure.

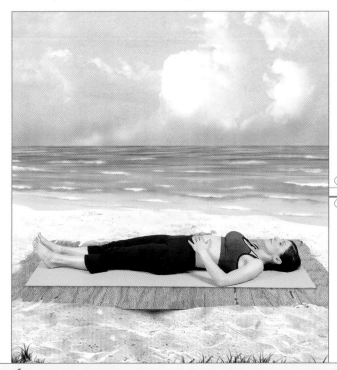
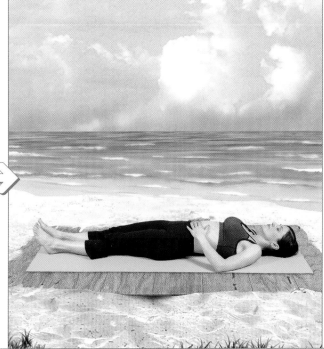

1 Begin in Relaxation Pose. For information on Relaxation Pose, see page 242.

2 Rest your palms lightly on your abdomen.

• The tips of your middle fingers should meet at your navel.

3 Inhale slowly and completely through your nose and feel your abdomen rise.

4 Exhale slowly and completely through your nose and feel your abdomen fall back down toward the floor.

5 Repeat steps 3 and 4 for 2 to 5 minutes.

three part breath *(dirgha pranayama)*

Three Part Breath exercise strengthens your chest, lung and diaphragm muscles, while increasing your lung capacity. Also called Full Yogic Breath or Complete Yoga Breath, practicing this exercise can also calm your mind and relax your body. You should be comfortable performing the abdominal breath exercise shown on page 37, before you try this exercise.

As you inhale in this exercise, focus on the expansion of your abdomen, ribs and then your chest. You may even be able to feel the movement of your breath up to your shoulders. As you exhale, feel these same areas fall, starting from your chest to your ribs and then to your abdomen. Your body should also soften and release as you exhale. Although you are breathing in three parts during this exercise, you should concentrate on taking one smooth inhalation and one smooth exhalation.

Use caution performing this exercise if you have serious lung or breathing problems.

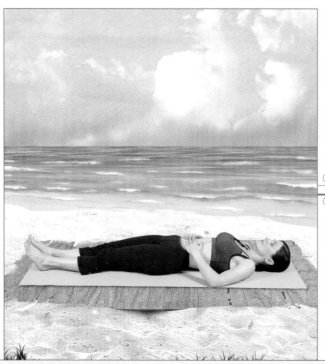

1 Begin in Relaxation Pose. For information on Relaxation Pose, see page 242.

2 Rest your palms lightly on your abdomen. The tips of your middle fingers should meet at your navel.

3 Inhale slowly through your nose and feel your abdomen rise.

4 Exhale slowly through your nose and feel your abdomen fall.

5 Repeat steps 3 and 4 until you feel comfortable breathing into your abdomen.

6 Rest your palms lightly on the bottom of your rib cage.

7 Inhale slowly through your nose and feel your rib cage expand.

8 Exhale slowly through your nose and feel your rib cage release.

9 Repeat steps 7 and 8 for three to five breaths.

How can I ensure that I am breathing correctly in this exercise?

You can use your arms as a guideline to ensure you are breathing correctly. As you inhale, raise your arms off the floor. When you feel the bottom of your ribs expand, your fingers should be pointing toward the ceiling. When you feel your chest expand, your arms should be on the floor above your head. Move your arms in the opposite direction as you exhale.

How can I feel more comfortable as I perform this exercise?

If your neck is tense, perform the exercise with a pillow or folded blanket under your head. If your back is uncomfortable, place a large pillow under your knees. You can also relieve strain on your back by bending your knees and placing your feet hip width apart on the floor.

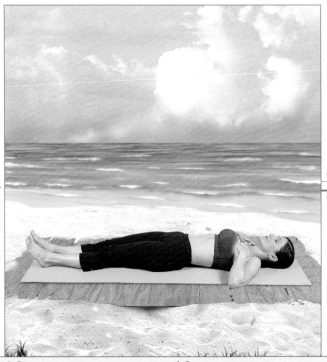

10 Rest your palms lightly on the top of your chest.

11 Inhale slowly through your nose and feel your chest expand.

12 Exhale slowly through your nose and feel your chest release.

13 Repeat steps 11 and 12 for three to five breaths.

14 Place one palm on your abdomen and place the other palm on your ribs or your chest.

15 Inhale slowly through your nose, feeling your abdomen, then your rib cage and then your chest expand.

16 Exhale slowly through your nose, allowing your breath to release from your chest, then your rib cage and then your abdomen.

17 Repeat steps 15 and 16 for 2 to 5 minutes.

Chapter 3

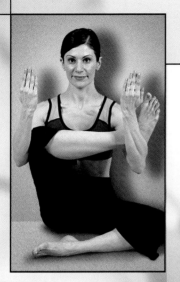

This chapter takes you through some warm-up exercises you can perform to prepare your body for a yoga practice. Warming up your muscles increases the flexibility of your joints, gets your blood circulating and loosens stiff muscles to help prevent injury. You should perform a warm-up sequence at the beginning of every yoga practice. You can include any of the poses discussed in this chapter in your own personalized warm-up sequence.

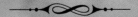

Warm-Up Poses

In this Chapter...

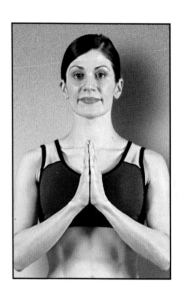

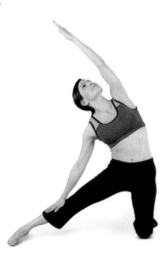

neck stretches

Neck stretching exercises are useful for warming up your neck and relaxing your neck, head and face. You may also find that neck stretches can relieve mental tension or stress that you may be experiencing.

You can perform neck stretches in a seated pose, such as Easy Pose or Lotus Pose. You can also perform neck stretches in a standing pose, such as Mountain Pose, or while sitting in a chair.

As you perform neck stretches, you should focus on sending your breath to the muscles in your neck that you want to relax. By focusing on your breath while stretching your neck, you can also help improve your awareness of your breathing as you practice yoga.

You should never feel any strain when stretching your neck. Make sure you only move your head to a position where you feel a comfortable stretch. You should also keep your jaw and shoulders relaxed throughout the exercise.

Use caution performing neck stretches if you have problems with your neck.

EXERCISE 1

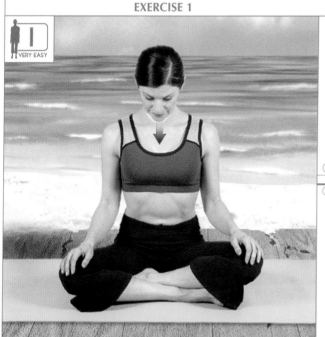 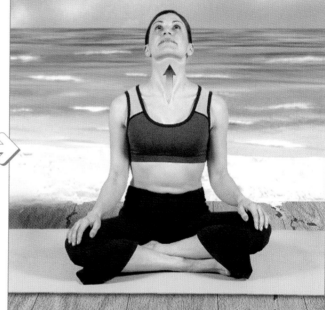

1 Begin in Easy Pose. For information on Easy Pose, see page 74.

2 Exhale and lower your chin toward your chest.
- Visualize the space you are creating in the back of your neck.

3 Inhale and raise your chin toward the ceiling.
- Visualize the front of your neck and throat gently stretching and opening.

- Make sure you keep the back of your neck long and do not allow your head to drop back.

4 Repeat steps 2 and 3 three to five times and then return your head to the center.

How can I provide a good stretch to the side of my neck?

With your chin parallel to the floor and the crown of your head pointing toward the ceiling, exhale and turn your head to look over your right shoulder. Then inhale and turn your head to look straight ahead. Repeat by looking over your left shoulder. Repeat three to five times on each side.

How can I release tension in my head and neck?

You can perform head rotations. Lower your chin to your chest and circle your head around to your right shoulder. Lift your head up, lower your head to your left shoulder and circle your head back down to your chest. Keep the back of your neck long as you rotate your head in a smooth, continuous movement. Repeat the head rotations two to three times and then switch directions.

EXERCISE 2

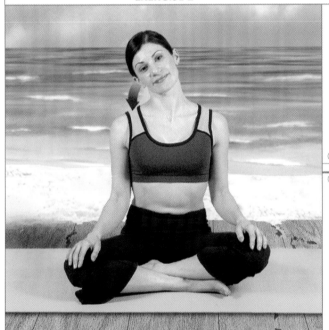

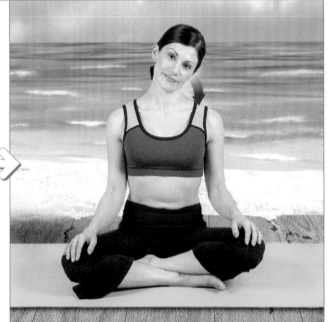

1 Begin in Easy Pose.

2 Exhale and lower your right ear toward your right shoulder.

• Make sure you keep your jaw and shoulders relaxed.

3 Inhale and return your head to an upright position.

4 Exhale and lower your left ear toward your left shoulder.

5 Inhale and return your head to an upright position.

6 Repeat steps 2 to 5 three to five times.

shoulder stretches

Shoulder stretching exercises are useful for relieving tightness in your upper back, shoulders and neck. You may also find that shoulder stretches can relieve stress and help clear your mind. Regular practice of shoulder stretches can increase the range of motion in your shoulders.

You can perform shoulder stretches in a seated pose, such as Easy Pose. You can also perform shoulder stretches in a standing pose, such as Mountain Pose, or while sitting in a chair.

As you perform the first exercise shown in the steps below, make sure you do not lift your shoulders. The stretch should only be a back and forward movement. The second exercise requires that you focus on the opposite movement. As you shrug your shoulders up and down, try not to move your shoulders forward or back. For both exercises, allow your arms to follow the movement of your shoulders, rather than participating in the stretch.

You should be careful performing shoulders stretches if you have a shoulder injury.

EXERCISE 1

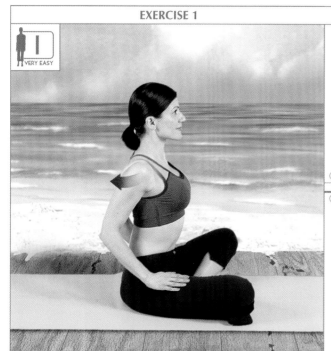 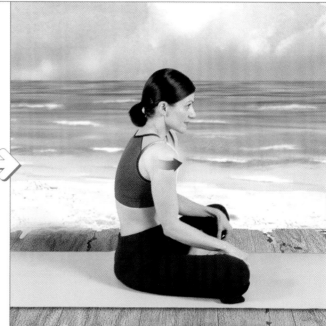

VERY EASY

1 Begin in Easy Pose. For information on Easy Pose, see page 74.

2 Inhale and squeeze your shoulders back, bringing your shoulder blades toward each other.
 • Visualize your chest opening and expanding.

3 Exhale and bring your shoulders forward, creating space between your shoulder blades.

 • Allow your arms to follow the movement of your shoulders.

4 Repeat steps 2 and 3 three to five times.

Is there an exercise that is particularly helpful for increasing the range of motion in my shoulders?

You can perform shoulder rolls. With your arms hanging loosely at your sides, make circles with your shoulders. Roll your shoulders backward three to five times. Then repeat rolling your shoulders forward. Make sure you maintain a fluid motion and keep your shoulders relaxed throughout the exercise.

How can I release tension in my upper back and neck?

You can perform a stretch that resembles giving yourself a hug. Bring your right arm across your chest and reach for your left shoulder blade. Then bring your left arm under your right arm and reach for your right shoulder blade. Tuck your chin toward your chest. With each exhalation, soften your shoulders, elbows and grip. Hold the stretch for 15 to 30 seconds and then repeat, switching the position of your arms.

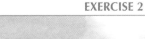

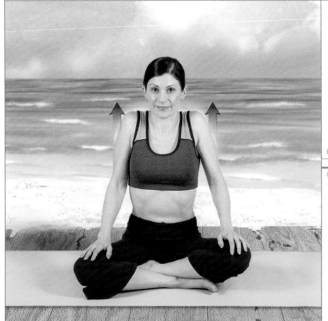

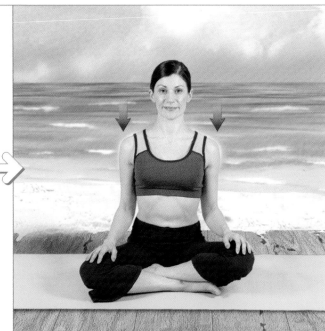

1 Begin in Easy Pose.

2 Inhale and lift your shoulders straight up toward your ears.

- Try to keep your shoulders from moving forward or back as you lift your shoulders up.

3 Exhale and slowly lower your shoulders back down.

- Make sure you control the movement of your shoulders. Do not allow your shoulders to simply drop down.

4 Repeat steps 2 and 3 three to five times.

arm stretches

Arm stretching exercises are an excellent way to warm up your arms in preparation for a yoga session. You can perform these exercises to improve the circulation in your upper body, particularly your arms, hands, fingers and the area around your heart. These exercises can also relieve tension from your shoulders and neck and even release tension from your mind.

The steps below illustrate two arm stretching exercises. As you perform the first exercise, your entire body should feel balanced. You should also focus on how your breathing works in connection with the arm movements to warm up your body and focus your mind.

As you perform these arm stretches, you should feel the lift coming from your waist as you raise your arms. At the same time, you should feel your chest lifting and expanding. Expanding your chest can increase your capacity for deep breathing in this exercise.

Make sure you use caution performing these arms stretches if you have shoulder or arm problems.

EXERCISE 1

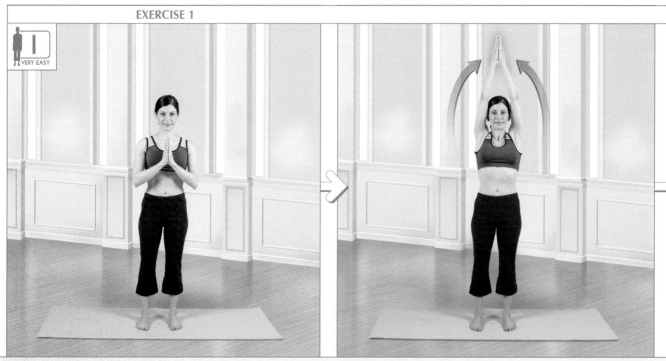

VERY EASY

1 Begin in Mountain Pose. For information on Mountain Pose, see page 120.

2 Position your hands in Prayer Pose. For information on Prayer Pose, see page 48.

3 Inhale as you circle your arms out to each side and then bring your palms together overhead.

- Your fingertips should be touching, with your fingers pointing toward the ceiling.

- Make sure your shoulders are relaxed down away from your ears.

- Your arms should be straight but your elbows should not be locked.

Is there an exercise I can perform to stretch the back of my upper arm?

To stretch the back of your upper arm, extend your right arm over your head. Then bend your right elbow and lightly rest your palm on the top of your right shoulder. Place your left palm slightly below your right elbow and gently press your right arm back until you feel the stretch. Then repeat this exercise for your other side.

Is there another arm stretch I can perform?

Yes. Interlace your fingers and extend your arms in front of you at shoulder level. Then turn your wrists so that your palms face out. Slowly raise your hands over your head. Gently straighten your arms as much as possible, but make sure you do not lock your elbows. You should feel the stretch from your waist up to your arms. Hold this stretch for 30 to 45 seconds.

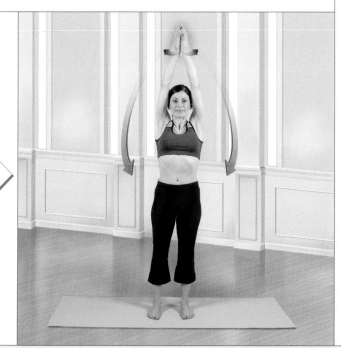

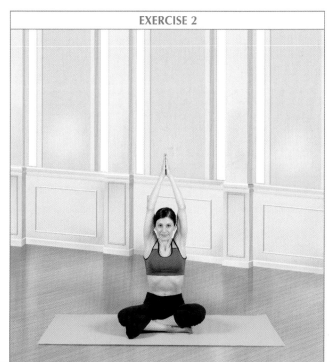

EXERCISE 2

4 Turn your palms to face out to the sides.

5 Exhale as you circle your arms out and down to each side and then bring your hands back together in Prayer Pose in front of your chest.

6 Repeat steps 3 to 5 three to five times.

1 Begin in Easy Pose. For information on Easy Pose, see page 74.

2 Rest the back of your hands on the floor at your sides.

3 Inhale as you raise your arms over your head, bringing your palms together.

4 Exhale and then lower your arms, bringing your hands back to the floor.

5 Repeat steps 3 and 4 three to five times.

prayer pose *(namaste)*

Prayer Pose is a basic arm position you can perform to create variety in many different standing or seated poses. This pose can help to increase the flexibility of your wrists.

While performing Prayer Pose, lift your chest as you roll your shoulders back and relax your shoulders and elbows down. Make sure you keep the pressure between your palms gentle and soft.

You can also perform Reverse Prayer Pose, which is very similar to Prayer Pose, except you position your hands behind your back. This pose stretches your shoulders and elbows, in addition to increasing the flexibility of your arms, wrists, hands and fingers.

In Reverse Prayer Pose, your hands should ideally be positioned between your shoulder blades, but only move your hands up as far as is comfortable for you. If you find this position too difficult, you can hold your elbows behind your back instead.

Use caution performing Prayer Pose or Reverse Prayer Pose if you have shoulder, arm or elbow problems.

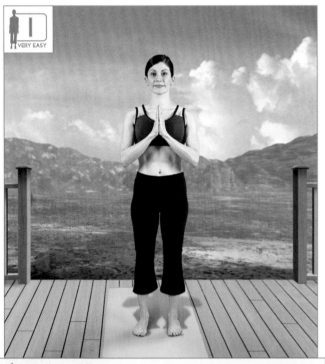

VERY EASY

1 Begin in Mountain Pose. For information on Mountain Pose, see page 120.

2 Bend your elbows and bring your palms together in front of the center of your chest.

• Your elbows should be lower than your wrists and your fingers should be pointing toward the ceiling.

3 Lift your chest toward your thumbs as you relax your shoulders down.

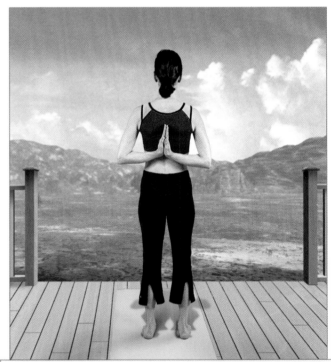

Reverse Prayer Pose

1 Begin in Mountain Pose.

2 Move your arms behind your back and bring your fingertips together, with your fingers pointing toward the floor.

3 Turn your hands inward until your fingers are pointing toward the ceiling.

4 Press your palms together and slowly move your hands up your back as far as is comfortable for you.

spinal roll

Spinal Roll is a great exercise to perform to warm up your spine. This exercise can also relieve tension in your lower back, which is especially useful if you spend a lot of time standing.

You can perform Spinal Roll as a transition from seated to standing poses. Spinal Roll is also useful for coming out of standing forward bends. Instead of coming out of a standing forward bend with a flat back, you can perform Spinal Roll which places less stress on your lower back. If you have lower back problems, coming

out of a standing forward bend with Spinal Roll is particularly helpful.

As you allow your upper body to hang down in Spinal Roll, visualize space being created between each vertebra of your spine as your spine lengthens toward the floor. As you roll up, focus on rolling your spine up one vertebra at a time—stacking each vertebra on top of the previous one.

Make sure you use caution performing Spinal Roll if you have high blood pressure.

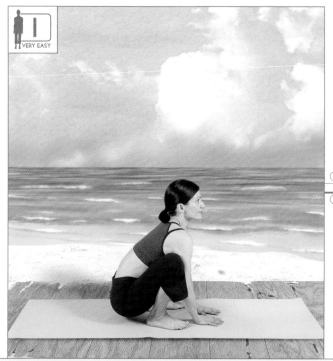
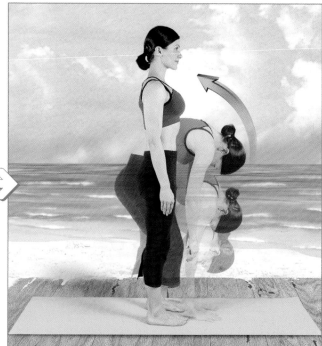

VERY EASY

1 Begin in Squat Pose. For information on Squat Pose, see page 68.

2 Place your hands on the floor slightly in front of you, with your palms facing down.

3 Press your hands into the floor.

4 Exhale as you straighten your legs, lifting your hips toward the ceiling.

5 Allow your hands to lift off the floor and your upper body to hang loosely toward the floor. Relax your head, neck and shoulders.

6 Press your feet into the floor and bend your knees slightly.

7 Tuck your tailbone under and inhale as you slowly roll your spine up one vertebra at a time.

• Your shoulders, neck and head should come up last.

spinal rocking

Spinal Rocking, also called Rocking Chair, is useful for massaging and warming up your spine. Massaging your spine helps relax your nervous system. You can perform Spinal Rocking to alleviate drowsiness or stiffness you may experience when you wake up in the morning. Spinal Rocking is also useful for warming up your spine for inversions, such as Shoulderstand shown on page 222.

Do not practice Spinal Rocking on a hard surface. Instead, spread a blanket the length of your body flat

out on the floor. Make sure that when you roll back, your head stays at the same level as your spine and does not roll off the edge of the blanket.

In the modified version of Spinal Rocking, you can hold the pose to stretch your upper back and neck. Make sure you avoid this modification if you have high blood pressure, a neck injury or if you are menstruating.

You should avoid Spinal Rocking if you have a neck, upper back or spinal injury.

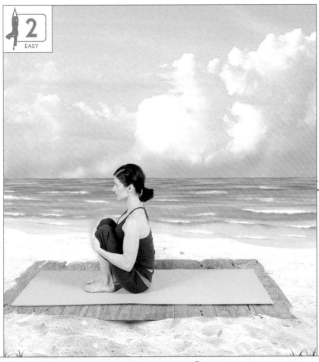

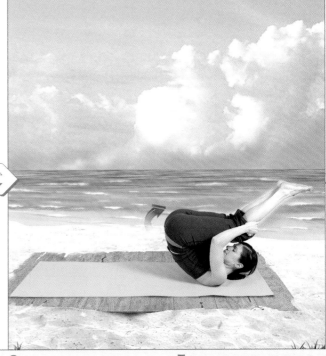

1 Sit on the floor with your knees bent, as close to your chest as possible.

• Your feet should be flat on the floor, hip width or slightly wider apart.

2 Hold your legs just below or behind your knees.

3 Tilt your head toward your chest to lengthen the back of your neck.

4 Keep your spine rounded as you exhale and roll backward.

5 Straighten your legs slightly as you roll back.

• Make sure you do not roll too far back on your neck.

How can I improve my balance as I perform Spinal Rocking?

To improve your balance, you can interlace your fingers behind your knees. This modification can offer more stability as you rock back and forth.

What should I do if I find Spinal Rocking uncomfortable?

If you would like to massage your spine, but find Spinal Rocking uncomfortable, you may want to perform Little Boat Pose instead. For information on massaging your spine in Little Boat Pose, see the top of page 59.

Can I move from Spinal Rocking into Plow Pose?

Yes. Spinal Rocking is a great way to move into Plow Pose. Perform the modification as described below, except straighten your legs and lower your feet toward the floor behind your head, with your feet flexed. For information on Plow Pose, see page 224.

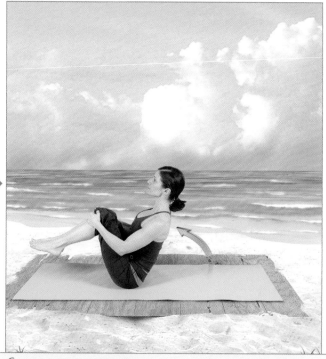

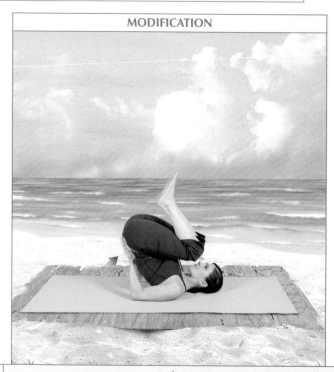

MODIFICATION

6 Inhale as you roll back up, bending your knees slightly.

7 As you roll up, press your shoulders down and back, lift your chest and chin up and look straight ahead.

- Make sure you lift out of the base of your spine to roll up.

- Visualize yourself gently rocking like a rocking chair.

8 Rock back and forth six to ten times.

- You can modify Spinal Rocking to stretch your upper back and neck.

1 When your shoulders reach the floor, place your elbows on the floor and place your hands on your lower back. Keep your knees bent and rest your thighs above your abdomen.

2 Hold the pose for 15 seconds to 1 minute.

rock the baby

Rock the Baby is a warm-up pose that provides an excellent stretch to your hips. You may want to perform this pose to prepare for seated poses, such as Half Lotus Pose or Lotus Pose. Rock the Baby is also a good stretch to perform in preparation for Lunge Pose.

As you rock your leg in this pose, make sure you focus on the movement in your hip, not the movement of your leg. It is also important to keep your spine as straight as possible in this stretch.

If you find it difficult to place your leg in the crooks of your elbows, you can perform the stretch with one hand holding your knee and one hand holding your ankle. You may also want to extend your other leg in front of you to help you stay grounded as you perform the stretch.

You should use caution performing Rock the Baby if you have knee or hip problems.

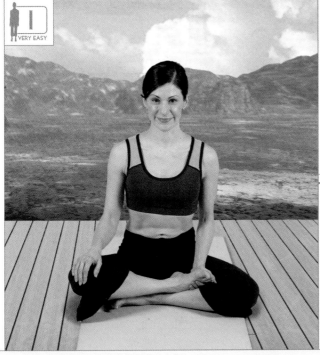

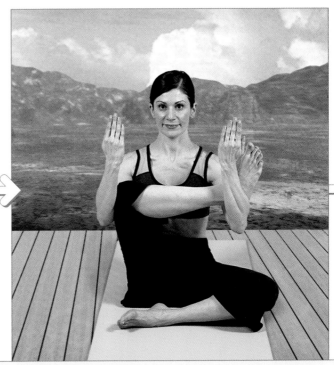

1 Begin in Easy Pose. For information on Easy Pose, see page 74.

2 Clasp your right foot with your left hand.

3 Clasp your right knee with your right hand.

4 Place your right foot in the crook of your left elbow.

5 Place your right knee in the crook of your right elbow.

- Your right shin should be parallel to the floor.

How can I increase the range of motion of my hips with Rock the Baby?

Clasp your right foot with your left hand and your right knee with your right hand and then circle your leg several times in each direction, making sure you do not pull on your knee. You should focus on the movement in your hip, not the movement of your knee. Repeat this movement using your other leg. This modification also helps to relieve tension in your hips.

Is there an easy way to perform Rock the Baby while at work?

Yes. You can perform Rock the Baby while sitting on a chair at work to help relieve any stiffness you may have in your hips. This is especially useful if you have been sitting in a chair all day long. Perform steps **2** to **10** below while sitting on a chair. Keep one foot on the floor as you rock your other leg and remember to keep your spine as straight as possible.

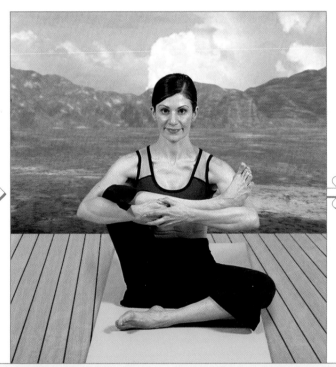

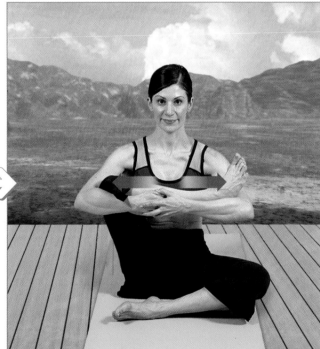

6 Wrap your arms around your right leg to support your leg.

- Keep your shoulders relaxed down away from your ears.

7 Press your sitting bones into the floor.

- Keep your spine as straight as possible.

8 Point the crown of your head toward the ceiling and gaze straight ahead.

9 Rock your right leg from side to side five to eight times. Then return to Easy Pose.

10 Repeat steps **2** to **9** for your other side.

- After performing Rock the Baby, you should shake out your legs to help relieve your hips, thighs, knees and ankles.

leg raises

Leg Raises warm up your legs and strengthen your abdominals and lower back. This exercise is also beneficial for stretching your hamstrings.

When you raise your leg in this exercise, your other leg may lift off the floor. Make sure that your other leg remains on the floor throughout the exercise. It is also important to make sure that you keep both of your hips on the floor throughout the exercise. To avoid arching your neck, you should lengthen your

neck by tucking your chin toward your chest.

Only raise your leg until you feel a comfortable stretch. It is more important to keep your lower back pressed into the floor and your shoulders relaxed down than it is to raise your leg as high as possible. Even if you are flexible, make sure you do not move your leg past a 90-degree angle with the floor.

You should use caution performing Leg Raises if you have problems with your neck or lower back.

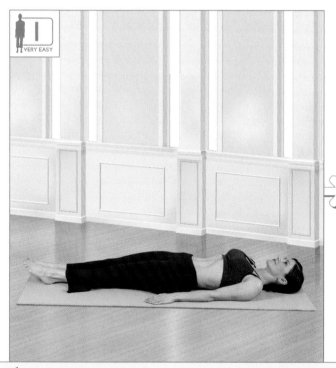

VERY EASY

1 Lie on your back with your legs extended and your feet together.

2 Place your arms on the floor at your sides, with your palms facing down.

• Your arms should be straight, but your elbows should not be locked.

3 Tuck your chin toward your chest to lengthen your neck.

• Your shoulders should be relaxed and down.

4 Exhale and press your lower back into the floor.

• Make sure your lower back remains pressed into the floor throughout the exercise.

What can I do to make this exercise easier?

To make Leg Raises easier, begin the exercise with one leg bent and the sole of your foot on the floor. Keep your foot on the floor as you raise and lower your other leg. This modification also helps to keep your lower back pressed into the floor, which protects your lower back from strain.

How can I make Leg Raises more challenging?

Once you feel comfortable raising one leg, you can perform the exercise raising both legs at the same time. As you perform this variation, remember to keep your lower back pressed into the floor and your shoulders relaxed. If you need extra support for your back, you can place your palms face down under your buttocks. Raise and lower your legs six to ten times. This variation makes the exercise more challenging for your abdominals and lower back.

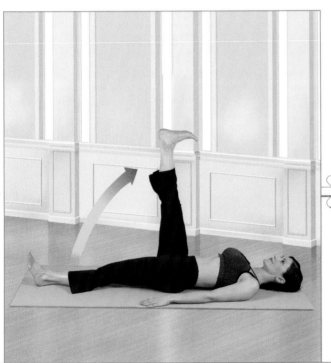

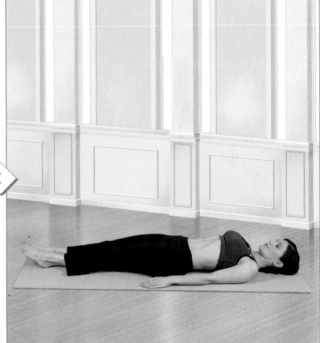

5 Flex your right foot.

6 Inhale and lift your right leg toward the ceiling.

- Keep your leg straight, but do not lock your knee as you raise your leg.

- Your leg should not move past a 90-degree angle with the floor.

7 Exhale and lower your right leg back down to the floor.

- As you lift and lower your leg, press through your heel and visualize your entire leg lengthening.

8 Repeat steps 6 and 7 three to eight times.

9 Repeat steps 1 to 8 for your other side.

pelvic tilt

Pelvic Tilt is a warm-up pose that increases the flexibility of your lower back and pelvis. The rocking movement of this pose also helps to lengthen your lower spine.

When you first perform Pelvic Tilt, you may be tempted to exaggerate the rocking motion of your pelvis. Instead, keep the movement of your pelvis natural and within your own range of motion. You should notice how the movement of your lower back creates a ripple effect up your spine. You should also try to coordinate the rocking motion with your breath and relax the muscles

that are not directly involved in the pose.

You can modify Pelvic Tilt by adding movement to your upper body as you rock your pelvis. Make sure you do not use your arms to lift your head and neck in this modification. You should keep your elbows back and your chest open, making sure you do not feel any strain in your neck.

Use caution performing Pelvic Tilt if you have slipped discs in your back.

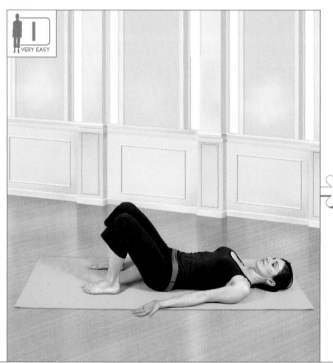

VERY EASY

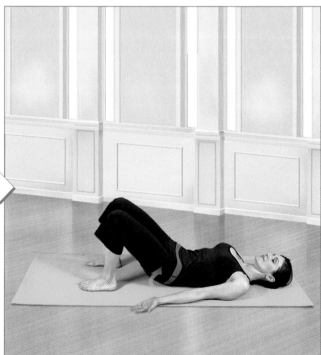

1 Lie on your back with your knees bent and your feet flat on the floor, hip width apart, with your heels directly under your knees.

2 Rest your arms on the floor at your sides, with your palms facing up.

3 Press out through the crown of your head to keep your neck long.

4 Exhale as you gently tilt your pelvis and press your lower back into the floor.

• As your pelvis tilts, your tailbone curls up and your hips remain on the floor.

I find coordinating my breath with my movement difficult. What can I do?

Although Pelvic Tilt is a breath awareness exercise, you may find coordinating your breath with your movement difficult. If this is a problem for you, try to focus only on the movement of your pelvis and breathe naturally. With time and practice, it will become easier to coordinate your breath and movement.

How can I further stretch my legs and strengthen my lower back in Pelvic Tilt?

Inhale as you tilt your pelvis and press your tailbone toward the floor. Then exhale as you tilt your pelvis and press your lower back into the floor. While maintaining this pelvic tilt, inhale as you press your feet into the floor and lift your pelvis off the floor. Then exhale as you curl your spine down one vertebra at a time. Repeat this movement three to six times.

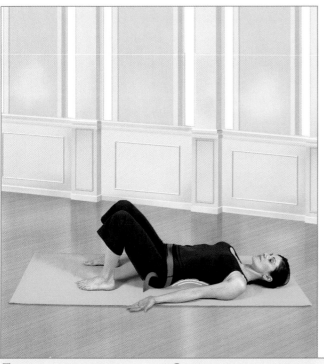

MODIFICATION

5 Inhale as you tilt your pelvis in the opposite direction and press your tailbone toward the floor.

• As your pelvis tilts, your lower back arches slightly.

6 Repeat steps 4 and 5 five to ten times to establish a gentle rocking motion of your pelvis.

• Visualize the rocking motion creating a ripple effect up your spine as you synchronize the motion with your breath.

• You can add upper body movement to Pelvic Tilt.

1 Perform Pelvic Tilt, except interlace your fingers behind your head. Your elbows should point out to the sides.

2 As you press your lower back into the floor, lift your chest, neck and head off the floor. Then lower your shoulders, neck and head back down as you arch your lower back.

3 Repeat this modification three to five times.

little boat pose *(pavana muktasana)*

Little Boat Pose stretches and releases your spine, lower back and hips. This pose is often used as a warm-up pose.

While performing Little Boat Pose, it is important to keep your arms and shoulders relaxed as you rest your hands on top of your knees. Do not use your arms to bring your knees toward your chest. Instead, release your hips so that your knees drop toward your chest naturally.

As you hold the pose, feel your body relaxing down to the floor with each exhalation. Visualizing yourself as a little boat bobbing on the waves of your breath may help you relax even further into the pose.

You can modify Little Boat Pose to release and stretch your hips independently. You can perform Little Boat Pose holding only one leg, while the other leg remains bent or stretched away from you. Do not stretch one leg away from you if you have lower back problems.

Avoid Little Boat Pose if you have recently had a hernia or a knee injury.

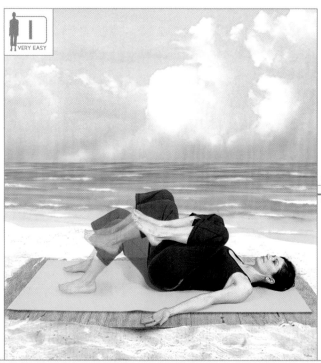

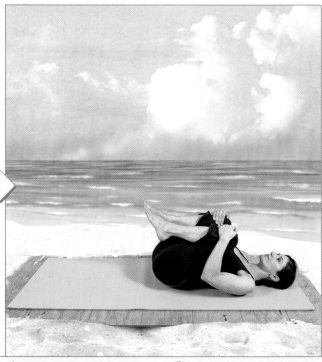

VERY EASY

1 Lie on your back with your knees bent and your feet flat on the floor, hip width apart.

2 Draw your knees toward your chest.

3 Release your lower back toward the floor.

4 Rest your hands on top of your knees. Your arms and shoulders should be relaxed.

5 Exhale as you relax your head, neck and spine toward the floor.

6 Soften and release your hips to allow your knees to drop further toward your chest.

7 Hold the pose for 30 seconds to 2 minutes.

Can I perform Little Boat Pose if I have stiff hips?

Yes. You can perform this pose if you have stiff hips, but you should move your knees wider than hip width apart when you draw them toward your chest. Widening your knees is also useful if you are overweight.

Resting my hands on top of my knees is uncomfortable. What else can I do?

You can wrap your arms around your legs or place your hands behind your knees in the area between your calf and thigh. In either variation, make sure you keep your arms and shoulders relaxed.

Can I add movement to Little Boat Pose?

To add movement to Little Boat Pose, perform the pose as described in the steps below and then rock your body from side to side. The rocking motion massages the back muscles on either side of your spine. This variation is particularly useful when you are using Little Boat Pose as a counter pose after performing a back bend.

MODIFICATION 1

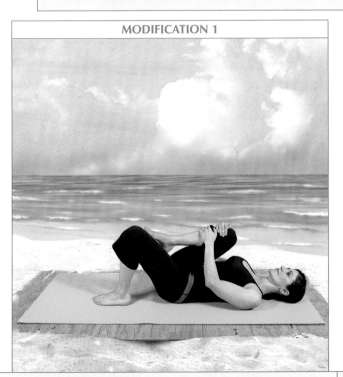

- You can perform Little Boat Pose holding one leg at a time. This allows you to stretch your hips independently.

1 Perform Little Boat Pose, except bring only your right knee toward your chest. Then repeat the modification for your other side.

MODIFICATION 2

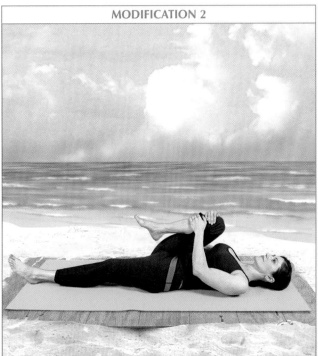

- You can perform Little Boat Pose holding one leg and stretching the other leg away from you. This allows you to feel a deeper stretch in your hips and lower back.

1 Perform Little Boat Pose, except start with your legs straight. Then bend your right knee and bring the knee toward your chest. Repeat the modification for your other side.

little boat twist *(parsva pavana muktasana)*

Little Boat Twist is beneficial for increasing the flexibility of your back and releasing tension in your lower and mid spine. This pose also helps to open your shoulders and chest. When you twist your body in Little Boat Twist, you stimulate your abdominal organs to help aid digestion. Although this pose is a useful warm-up pose, you may also want to use the pose to cool down at the end of a yoga practice.

While performing Little Boat Twist, make sure you keep your upper back and both shoulders in contact with the floor. You should also breathe evenly, visualizing your body softening deeper into the twist with each exhalation.

If you find the twist in Little Boat Twist too intense, you can perform the pose with your feet on the floor, instead of drawing your knees into your chest. Avoid performing Little Boat Twist if you have abdominal problems or if your neck feels strained in the pose.

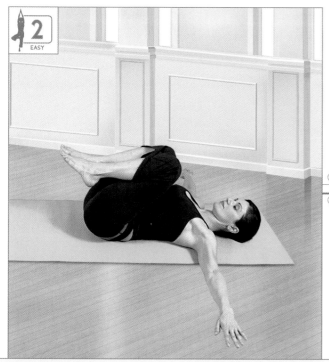

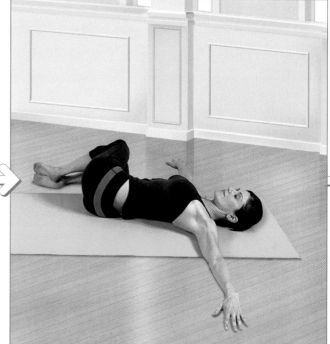

1 Begin in Little Boat Pose. For information on Little Boat Pose, see page 58.

2 Extend your arms out to your sides at shoulder height, with your palms facing down.

3 Exhale as you lower your knees to the right toward the floor. Keep your knees together.

• Make sure you keep your upper back and both shoulders in contact with the floor throughout the pose.

How can I incorporate movement into Little Boat Twist?

Perform the pose as described below, except slowly twist from side to side five to ten times instead of holding the pose. To coordinate your breathing with the movement, exhale as you move into the twist and inhale as your knees and head come back to the center. This movement helps massage your back and release tension in your spine.

How can I intensify the pose?

You can intensify the pose to provide a deeper stretch for your spine, lower back and hips. Perform the pose as described below, except after you lower your knees toward the floor, straighten your legs. Your upper body and legs should form a 90-degree angle. Make sure you keep your legs together and straight, but do not lock your knees.

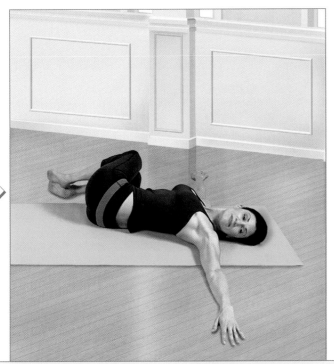

MODIFICATION

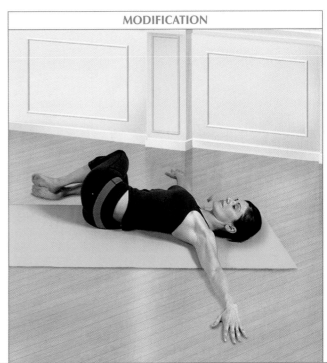

4 Turn your head to the left and look over your left shoulder, keeping your neck relaxed.

5 Hold the pose for 30 seconds to 1 minute and then inhale as you return to Little Boat Pose.

6 Repeat steps 2 to 5 for your other side.

• You can modify Little Boat Twist if you feel discomfort in your neck or shoulders.

1 If you feel discomfort in your neck, look up at the ceiling and tilt your chin slightly down to lengthen the back of your neck.

• If you feel discomfort in your shoulders, place your hands on the floor, with your palms facing up, and relax your shoulders down to the floor.

windmill pose

Windmill Pose is a reclined warm-up pose that helps to improve digestion and elimination. This pose also stretches your lower back and helps to strengthen your abdominal muscles. Windmill Pose is also known as Wind-Relieving Pose because it helps the body release intestinal gas.

You should focus on stretching the entire length of your body in Windmill Pose. The movement of your legs should help to increase the flexibility of your hips. At the same time, the movement massages the organs

in the back of your body, including your kidneys.

While performing Windmill Pose, make sure your hips remain on the floor throughout the pose. You should also pay close attention to your breathing—inhale as you stretch your arm and leg away from your body and exhale as you draw your arm and leg back to your body.

You should avoid Windmill Pose if you have a hernia.

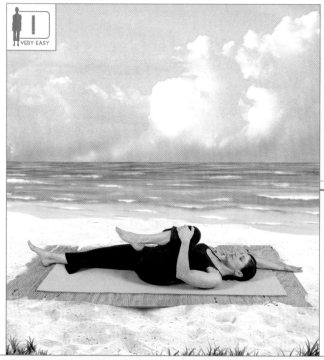

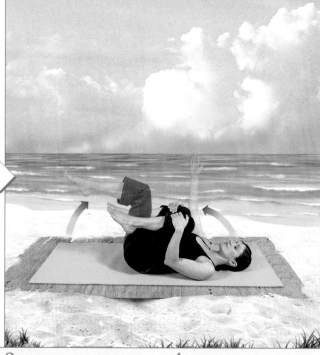

1 Begin in Little Boat Pose. For information on Little Boat Pose, see page 58.

2 Inhale as you raise your right arm overhead and extend your right leg along the floor.

• The back of your right hand and the heel of your right foot should touch the floor.

3 Exhale as you bring your right knee toward your chest and your right hand to your right knee.

4 Clasp your right knee with your right hand.

• Make sure your elbow remains close to your body.

How can I intensify the stretch in this pose?

When you clasp each knee, hold your knee for 5 to 10 seconds. You should exhale as you draw your knee in and inhale as you extend your leg out.

What can I do if my lower back feels strained in this pose?

You can begin the pose with your knees bent and the soles of your feet resting on the floor. Keep one foot on the floor as you bring the other knee to your chest.

How can I stretch my neck and shoulders in this pose?

When you bring your knee toward your chest, move your forehead toward your knee. In this modification, make sure you do not strain your neck or shoulders trying to reach your forehead to your knee.

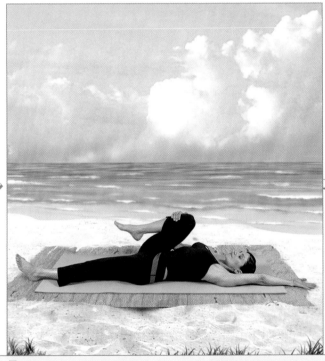

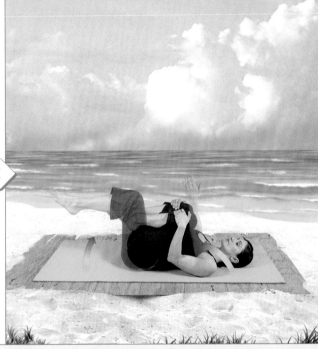

5 Inhale as you raise your left arm overhead and extend your left leg along the floor.

• The back of your left hand and the heel of your left foot should touch the floor.

6 Exhale as you bring your left knee toward your chest and your left hand to your left knee.

7 Clasp your left knee with your left hand.

8 Repeat steps 2 to 7 six or eight times.

9 To come out of the pose, place the soles of your feet on the floor and bring your arms to rest alongside your body.

gate pose *(parighasana)*

Gate Pose is an invigorating pose that provides a good stretch to the sides of your body and increases the flexibility of your spine. You can also use this pose to tone your abdominal muscles and improve your circulation. Gate Pose is an excellent pose to perform in preparation for Triangle Pose. While both poses stretch similar muscles, Gate Pose does not require the intense stretch to the back of your legs.

Performing Gate Pose stretches the muscles that connect your ribs, allowing your lungs to expand to help increase your capacity for deep breathing. As a result, practicing this pose is especially useful if you have a breathing problem, such as asthma.

While performing Gate Pose, make sure your elbow does not move in front of your face, but stretches up above your ear. You should also focus on lengthening your spine with each inhalation and stretching to your side with each exhalation.

Use caution performing this pose if you suffer from knee, hip or shoulder problems.

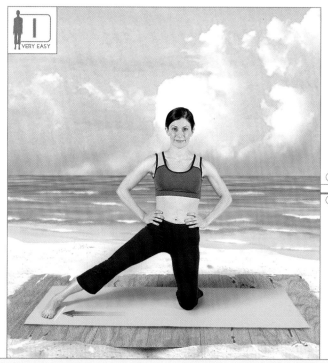

VERY EASY

1 Kneel on the floor with your knees hip width apart and your thighs parallel.

2 Extend your right leg to your right side.

3 Place the sole of your right foot flat on the floor, with your toes pointing forward.

• Your right leg should be straight, but your knee should not be locked.

4 Rest your right hand on the outside of your right thigh.

5 Inhale and extend your left arm overhead, with your fingers pointing toward the ceiling and your palm facing your right side.

• Your left upper arm should remain beside your left ear throughout the pose.

I feel pressure on my knees in this pose. What can I do?

To reduce the pressure on your knees, you can perform the pose while kneeling on a blanket or mat.

My neck feels uncomfortable when I look up past my elbow. Can I still perform the pose?

You can still perform this pose, but you should look straight ahead instead of turning your head to look past your elbow.

How can I stretch my foot and the back of my calf more in Gate Pose?

Instead of placing the sole of your foot flat on the floor, place your heel on the floor with your toes pointing up toward the ceiling. This modification also provides a deeper stretch to your hamstring.

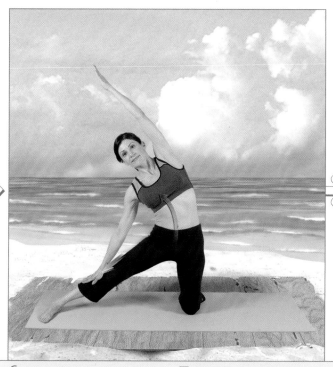

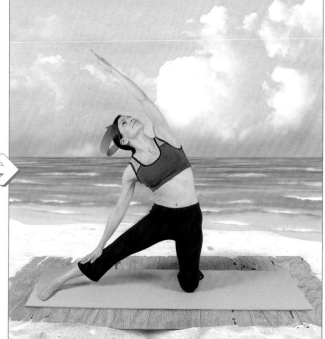

6 Exhale and bend from the waist as you stretch to the right.

- Keep your left shoulder back and relaxed as you stretch to the right.

7 Slide your right hand down the outside of your right leg.

- Your right arm should be straight, but your elbow should not be locked.

8 Turn your head to look past your left elbow.

9 Press your right foot into the floor as you extend out through your fingertips and the crown of your head.

10 Hold the pose for 10 to 20 seconds.

11 To come out of the pose, inhale and bring your torso upright. Then exhale and bring your arms to your sides and your knees together.

12 Repeat steps 2 to 11 for your other side.

pigeon pose *(kapotasana)*

Pigeon Pose helps to open and increase the flexibility of your hips. This pose also helps to strengthen your back, stretch your thighs and increase the flexibility of your groin.

Practicing this pose may help you perform other poses that require a lot of flexibility in your hips, such as Lotus Pose and Dancer Pose. You may also want to use Pigeon Pose to warm up before performing back bends, such as Cobra Pose and Bow Pose.

As you perform Pigeon Pose, make sure you gently press the hip of your straight leg toward the floor to help keep your hips square to the front. Hold the pose for as long as you feel comfortable, allowing yourself to relax further into the pose with each exhalation. After performing the pose, you should shake out your legs to help relieve and restore circulation in your legs.

You should use caution performing Pigeon Pose if you have problems with your knees, back or hips.

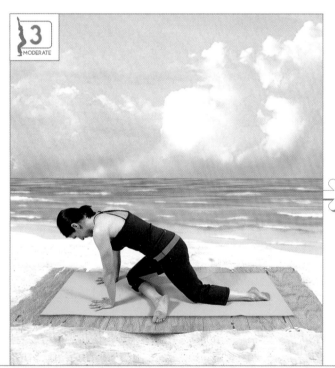

1 Begin in Table Pose. For information on Table Pose, see page 172.

2 Slide your right knee forward, under the center of your body.

3 Bring your right foot to the left side of your body.

• You can rest your right foot underneath your pubic bone or out to your left side.

4 Slide your left leg straight behind you. The top of your left foot should rest on the floor.

5 Gently lower your pelvis toward the floor.

• Make sure you keep both hips square to the front.

• If your right hip cannot reach the floor, you can place a folded blanket under your hip for support.

My forehead is uncomfortable in this pose. What can I do?

If you find resting your forehead on the floor uncomfortable, you can bend your elbows and place one hand on top of the other. Then rest your forehead on your hands.

How can I modify Pigeon Pose to help release tension in my hips?

To help release tension in your hips, you can rock your hips from side to side as you hold the pose.

How can I make this pose more challenging?

To make Pigeon Pose more challenging, perform the pose as described below, except when you lower your elbows to the floor, position your elbows directly below your shoulders, press your forearms into the floor and lift your chest toward the ceiling. As you become more comfortable in this position, you can gradually straighten your arms and move your hands closer to your body to lift your chest up further.

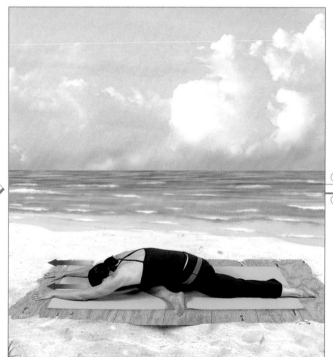

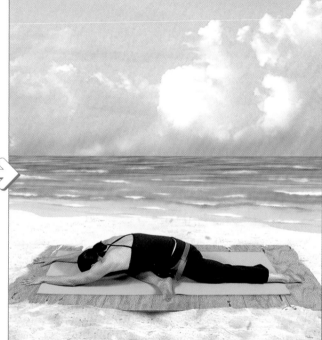

6 Slide your hands forward along the floor and lower your elbows to the floor.

7 Continue sliding your hands until your arms are straight, but your elbows are not locked.

8 Exhale as you lower your chest toward the floor.

9 Rest your forehead on the floor.

10 Gently press your left hip toward the floor to help keep your hips square.

11 Hold the pose for 15 seconds to 1 minute.

• To come out of the pose, slide your hands back under your shoulders and return to Table Pose.

12 Repeat steps 2 to 11 for your other side.

squat pose

Squat Pose helps to open your hips, groin and inner thighs, while stretching your ankles and feet. This pose can also relieve tension in your lower back. Regular practice of Squat Pose can help improve your balance and concentration.

This pose is commonly used as a transition from seated to standing poses. From a seated pose, you can move into Squat Pose and then slowly roll your spine up, one vertebra at a time, to a standing position. Squat Pose is

also a good prenatal exercise because it stimulates your pelvic area and opens your groin and hips.

To help you balance and feel more comfortable in the pose, you may need to adjust your stance after you bend your knees and lower your hips. You may find it helpful to move your feet a bit further apart or turn your toes out slightly.

Use caution performing Squat Pose if you have problems with your knees or hips.

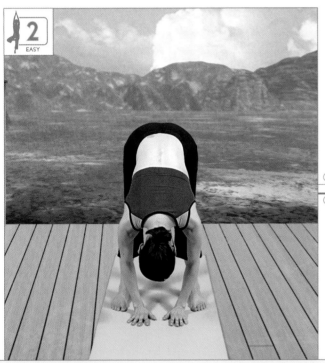

1 Begin in Mountain Pose. For information on Mountain Pose, see page 120.

2 Step your feet slightly wider than hip width apart, with your toes pointing forward.

3 Bend forward from your hips.

4 Place your hands on the floor slightly in front of you, with your palms facing down.

5 Keeping your hands on the floor for support, bend your knees and lower your hips toward the floor.

6 Gently lower your heels toward the floor.

7 Move your elbows or upper arms to the inside of your knees and then bring your hands together in Prayer Pose. For information on Prayer Pose, see page 48.

My heels do not reach the floor when I perform Squat Pose. What can I do?

If your heels do not reach the floor, you can remain on the balls of your feet, or place a rolled or folded blanket under your heels for support. Make sure the blanket is not so thick that it pushes your heels up further. The blanket should only support your heels at the lowest position possible.

What can I do if I find it difficult to balance in this pose?

You can leave your hands on the floor for support instead of bringing your hands together in Prayer Pose. You can also move into Squat Pose with your back against a wall for support. Slowly slide your back down the wall to lower your hips into the pose. As you slide down, allow your heels to lift off the floor.

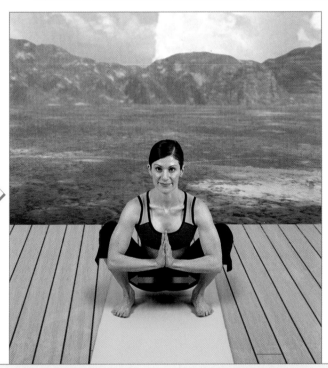

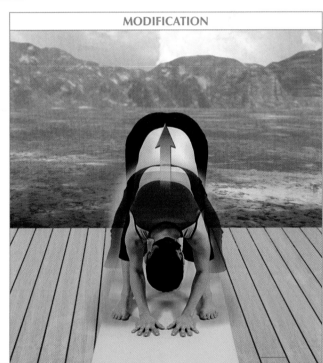

MODIFICATION

8 Gently press your elbows or upper arms against your inner legs to open your hips, inner thighs and groin.

9 Point the crown of your head toward the ceiling.

10 Hold the pose for 30 seconds to 1 minute.

11 To come out of the pose, bring your hands back to the floor, straighten your legs and then roll your spine up, one vertebra at a time. Then return to Mountain Pose.

• You can add motion to Squat Pose to energize your spine.

1 Perform Squat Pose, except keep your hands on the floor instead of placing your hands in Prayer Pose.

2 Inhale as you lift your hips toward the ceiling and move the crown of your head toward the floor. Then exhale and lower your hips back toward the floor.

3 Lift and lower your hips ten times.

Chapter 4

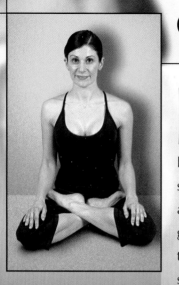

Performing seated poses can improve your posture, stretch your legs and open your hips. Some seated poses, such as Easy Pose and Lotus Pose, are especially good for meditation because they allow you to keep your spine straight and help you remain grounded and relaxed as you meditate. Certain seated poses are often used as starting positions for other poses. This chapter demonstrates a variety of seated poses that you can perform.

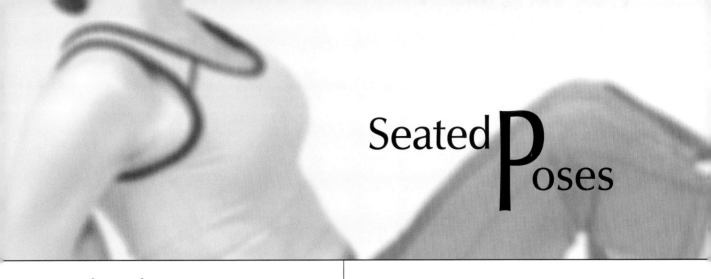

Seated Poses

In this Chapter...

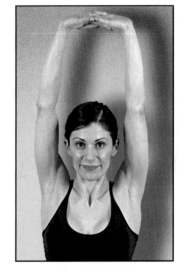

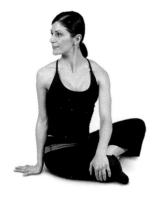

staff pose *(dandasana)*

Staff Pose can help you learn how to sit with correct posture. Regular practice of this pose can also help increase the flexibility of your hips and pelvis and strengthen your lower back. This basic seated pose often serves as a starting position for other seated poses.

While you perform Staff Pose, you should be aware of both your upper and lower body. Your upper body should be erect, yet relaxed, and your lower body should feel grounded.

To provide extra support for your spine in this pose, you can place your palms directly behind your body with your fingers pointing behind you, instead of placing your palms beside your hips. If your hips are stiff, you can perform the pose sitting on a folded blanket. This modification raises your hips so your legs drop away from your pelvis, allowing you to sit more comfortably. Sitting on a folded blanket may also help keep you from rounding your lower back and can make finding the correct alignment of your spine easier.

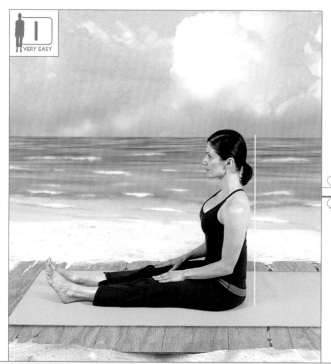

VERY EASY

1 Sit on the floor with your back straight and your legs stretched out in front of you.

• Make sure your legs and feet are hip width apart and parallel.

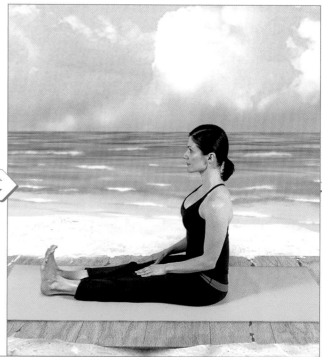

2 Press your sitting bones into the floor and point the crown of your head toward the ceiling to lengthen and straighten your spine.

3 Flex your feet and press out through your heels.

How can I modify Staff Pose if I have back problems?

If you have back problems or find this pose difficult to hold, you can perform the pose with your back lightly touching a wall. You can also choose to perform Legs Up the Wall Pose, which will protect your back even more while still providing the benefits of Staff Pose. For information on Legs Up the Wall Pose, see page 218.

How can I stretch my upper body in Staff Pose?

To stretch your upper body in Staff Pose, interlace your fingers and then extend your arms forward, parallel to the floor. Turn your palms away from you so your thumbs are pointing toward the floor and then inhale as you raise your arms above your head until your arms are positioned slightly behind your ears. Be sure to keep your shoulders relaxed as you perform this variation. Stretching your upper body in Staff Pose can help open your chest and stretch the front of your abdomen.

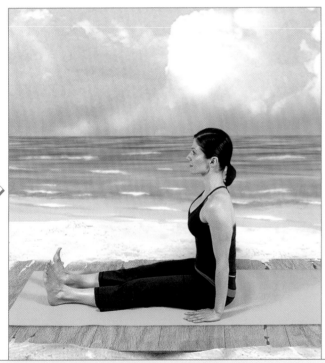

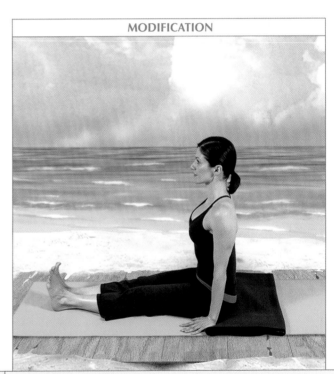

MODIFICATION

4 Place your palms on the floor beside your hips to support your spine and then relax your shoulders down. Your upper body should be erect, but relaxed.

5 Relax your legs to the floor so your lower body feels firmly grounded.

6 Hold the pose for 20 to 30 seconds.

1 If you have stiff hips, perform Staff Pose sitting on a folded blanket.

• Sitting on a folded blanket raises your hips so your legs drop away from your pelvis, allowing you to sit more comfortably. This modification can also help you lengthen and straighten your spine more easily.

easy pose *(sukhasana)*

Easy Pose is a calming pose that is useful for meditation and practicing breathing exercises. This pose also helps to promote proper seated posture.

Each time you perform Easy Pose, you should alternate which leg you place on top. While performing the pose, allow the crown of your head to lift up as your spine elongates and press your sitting bones down into the floor. You should focus on keeping your spine straight in this pose.

While performing Easy Pose, focus on moving your breath through your body. You may find closing your eyes helps you relax into the pose. You can hold the pose for as long as you need to calm your mind.

If your hips are stiff or your knees are strained, try sitting on thickly folded blankets. Sitting on blankets can also help prevent you from rounding your lower back or raising your knees up higher than your pelvis. Even with this modification, use caution performing Easy Pose if you have problems with your knees or hips.

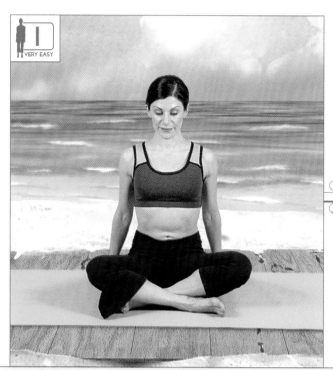

VERY EASY

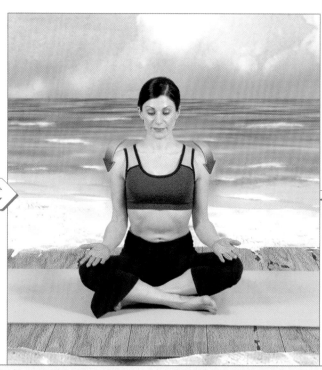

1 Begin in Staff Pose. For information on Staff Pose, see page 72.

2 Bend your knees and cross your legs in front of you.

3 Draw your feet toward your buttocks as far as is comfortable for you.

4 Place your hands on your knees with your palms facing up.

5 Relax your shoulders down and back, and lift and expand your chest.

6 Press your sitting bones toward the floor and lengthen your spine.

How can I support my back while performing Easy Pose?

To provide support for your back in this pose, perform the pose sitting with your back lightly touching a wall. The wall can act as a guideline for your spine to help prevent you from rounding your lower back and shoulders.

What should I do if my feet are sore in Easy Pose?

If your feet are sore, you can place a folded towel or blanket under your feet. This can help relieve pressure on your feet.

Is there another variation of Easy Pose?

Yes. You can perform Easy Pose without crossing your legs. Instead, bend one knee so the outside of your leg is resting on the floor. Then draw your foot toward your buttock as far as is comfortable for you. Bend your other knee and rest the outside of your leg on the floor so your heel is just in front of the shin of your other leg.

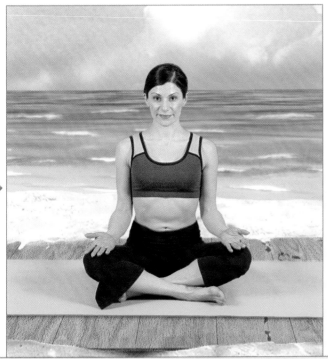

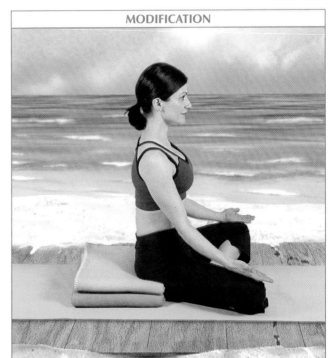

MODIFICATION

7 Point the crown of your head toward the ceiling and gaze straight ahead.

8 Hold the pose for 1 to 10 minutes. Then return to Staff Pose.

• After performing Easy Pose, you should shake out your legs to help relieve your knees and ankles.

1 If your hips are stiff or if you have discomfort in your knees, you can perform Easy Pose sitting on the edge of two or three thickly folded blankets. This allows your knees to drop so you can sit straight more easily.

bound angle pose *(baddha konasana)*

Bound Angle Pose provides a stretch to your groin and inner thighs. You can also use this pose to develop flexibility in your hips, knees, ankles and feet.

Practicing Bound Angle Pose opens the front of your pelvis and promotes circulation in your pelvic floor. For these reasons, this pose is often used as a prenatal exercise and is helpful for relieving menstrual problems.

While performing Bound Angle Pose, make sure you rest your weight on your sitting bones as you drop

your knees toward the floor. You should feel a stretch, but no pain, in your knees. If your knees are high up off the floor, do not force them down. Instead, move your feet further away from your groin or place rolled up blankets under your knees for support. After you come out of Bound Angle Pose, you should perform Staff Pose or shake out your legs to relieve your knees and ankles.

You should avoid Bound Angle Pose if you have a knee or groin injury.

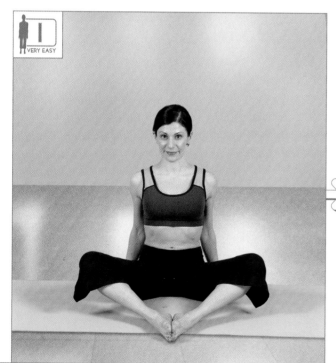

VERY EASY

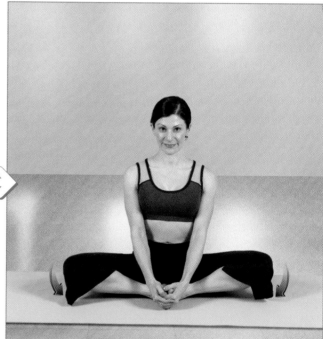

1 Begin in Staff Pose. For information on Staff Pose, see page 72.

2 Bend your legs and place the soles of your feet together.

3 Clasp your feet or ankles and then move your heels toward your groin as far as is comfortable for you.

4 Exhale as you allow your knees to drop toward the floor.

5 Relax your shoulders and arms.

How can I incorporate movement into Bound Angle Pose?

To incorporate movement into Bound Angle Pose, gently bounce your knees up and down as you perform the pose. This variation, called Butterfly Pose, helps to further release tension from your groin area and open your hips and inner thighs. When performing this variation, visualize your knees moving like the wings of a butterfly.

How can I relieve tightness in my hips while performing Bound Angle Pose?

Perform the pose as described below and then rock your body from side to side. The rocking motion massages your hips to relieve tightness and tension. This variation of Bound Angle Pose is also useful as a warm-up in preparation for other poses.

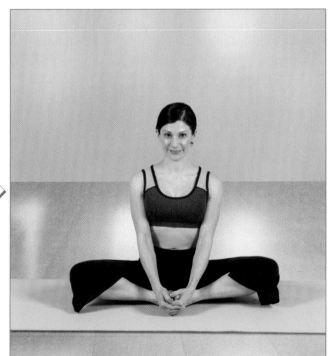

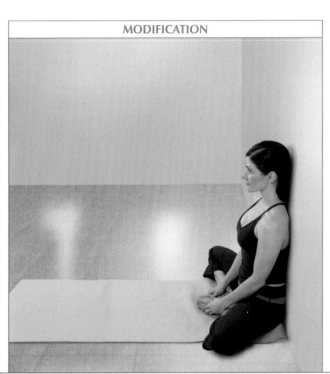

MODIFICATION

6 Press your sitting bones into the floor and point the crown of your head toward the ceiling to lengthen your spine.

• Visualize your knees opening like the wings of a butterfly.

7 Hold the pose for 30 seconds to 2 minutes and then return to Staff Pose.

• You can perform Bound Angle Pose with your back touching a wall. This is useful if you have a weak lower back and require extra support.

1 Perform Bound Angle Pose, except sit with your back lightly touching a wall.

half lotus pose *(ardha padmasana)*

Half Lotus Pose is a seated pose that stretches and helps to open your hips. This pose is also useful for practicing breathing exercises and meditation. To warm up for Half Lotus Pose, you can perform Rock the Baby, as shown on page 52.

While Performing Half Lotus Pose, you should try to keep your knees as close to the floor as possible. You can place a thickly folded blanket under your raised knee for support if your knee feels strained in this

pose. Make sure you come out of the pose if you feel any pain in your knees.

You can change the position of your hands to create variety in the pose. For example, you can rest the back of your hands on your thighs with the tips of your thumbs and first fingers touching or you can position your hands in Prayer Pose, as shown on page 48.

Use caution performing Half Lotus Pose if you have knee or hip problems.

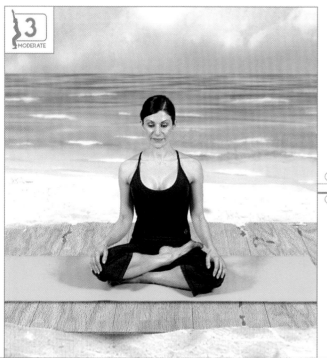
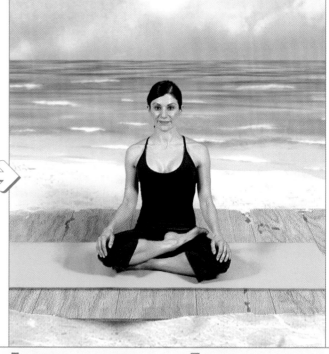

1 Begin in Staff Pose. For information on Staff Pose, see page 72.

2 Bend your right leg and place your right foot on your left thigh, as close to your hip as possible.

3 Bend your left leg and slide your left foot under your right leg.

4 Rest your palms on your thighs.

5 Exhale as you press your sitting bones into the floor and point the crown of your head toward the ceiling.

6 Hold the pose for 5 seconds to 1 minute or as long as is comfortable for you. Then return to Staff Pose.

7 Repeat steps 2 to 6 for your other side.

• After performing Half Lotus Pose, you should shake out your legs to help relieve your knees and ankles.

lotus pose *(padmasana)*

Lotus Pose is an intermediate to advanced seated pose that provides a deep stretch for your hips. This pose can also help to open your hips and improve your seated posture. You may want to use this pose for breathing exercises or meditation.

You should feel comfortable performing Half Lotus Pose, as shown on page 78, before you try Lotus Pose. You can also perform Pigeon Pose or Bound Angle Pose to help prepare you for Lotus Pose.

To help relieve pressure in your knees in this pose, you can sit on a thickly folded blanket. Sitting on a blanket will also support your pelvis and help prevent your lower back from rounding. If you feel any pain in your knees, you should come out of the pose.

To help you relax in this pose, close your eyes and visualize yourself as the lotus flower, with your roots holding you firmly in the ground while you bloom in the sunshine.

Use caution performing Lotus Pose if you have knee or hip problems.

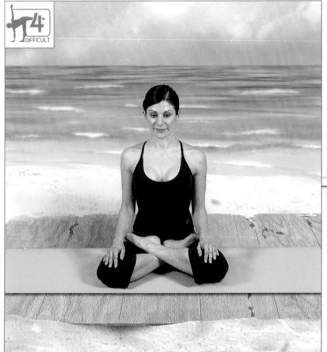

1 Begin in Staff Pose. For information on Staff Pose, see page 72.

2 Bend your right leg and place your right foot on your left thigh, as close to your hip as possible.

3 Bend your left leg and place your left foot on your right thigh, as close to your right hip as possible.

4 Rest your palms on your thighs.

5 Exhale as you press your sitting bones into the floor and point the crown of your head toward the ceiling.

6 Hold the pose for 5 seconds to 1 minute or as long as is comfortable for you. Then return to Staff Pose.

7 Repeat steps 2 to 6 bending your left leg first.

• After performing Lotus Pose, you should shake out your legs to help relieve your knees and ankles.

cow face pose *(gomukhasana)*

Cow Face Pose is an uplifting pose that provides a good stretch for your arms and shoulders. This pose is also beneficial for releasing tension in your shoulders and opening your chest to help facilitate deep breathing. If you have rounded shoulders, you can perform Cow Face Pose to help improve your posture.

While performing Cow Face Pose, try to keep both sitting bones on the floor and your knees stacked on top of each other. The position of your legs in this pose provides a great stretch for your hips, thighs and ankles.

When you clasp your hands behind your back in this pose, remember to keep your shoulders square to the front and your chest expanded. Make sure you do not hunch your shoulders or twist your wrists to clasp your hands.

Use caution performing Cow Face Pose if you have shoulder problems, such as rotator cuff tendonitis. You should also be careful performing this pose if you have neck, hip or knee problems.

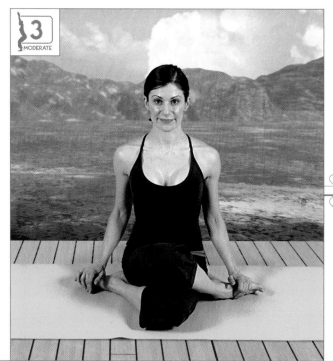

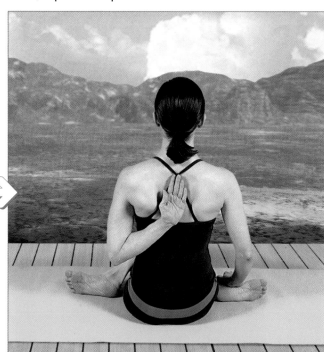

1 Begin in Staff Pose. For information on Staff Pose, see page 72.

2 Bend your left leg and bring your left heel under your right thigh, near your right hip.

3 Bend your right leg over your left knee and bring your right heel near your left hip.

• Make sure your right knee is directly above your left knee.

4 Rest your palms on your feet.

5 Press your sitting bones into the floor and point the crown of your head toward the ceiling to lengthen your spine.

6 Bend your left elbow and bring your left forearm behind your back.

7 Rest the back of your left hand in the middle of your back, near your shoulder blades.

• Your left forearm and the fingers of your left hand should be pointing toward your head.

What can I do if I cannot clasp my hands behind my back?

You can hold a strap with your hands as close together as is comfortable for you. Then gently pull your elbows away from each other.

What should I do if I find the leg position in this pose too difficult?

You can perform the upper body stretch of this pose while sitting in Easy Pose, as shown on page 74, or Thunderbolt Pose, as shown on page 90.

How can I deepen the pose?

Before you hold the pose, pull your abdominal muscles toward your spine and bend forward from your hips as you gently press your chest toward the floor. Make sure you keep your hands clasped and your elbows pulling away from each other. This modification helps to relieve headaches and also allows you to breathe through your nose more easily.

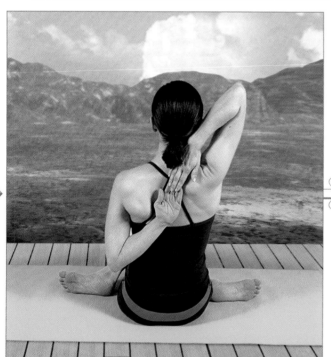

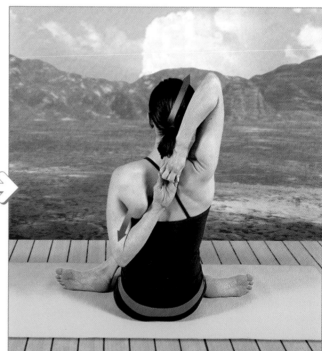

8 Inhale and extend your right arm over your head.

9 Bend your right elbow and place your right hand between your shoulder blades.

• Your right palm should be facing your back and the fingers of your right hand should be pointing toward the floor.

10 With your right hand, clasp the fingers of your left hand.

11 Gently pull your elbows away from each other. Feel your shoulders stretching and your chest opening.

12 Hold the pose for 10 to 30 seconds and then release your hands and return to Staff Pose.

13 Repeat steps 2 to 12 for your other side.

seated side bend

Seated Side Bend stretches the sides of your body, from your hips to your fingertips.

While performing Seated Side Bend, remember that it is more important to lengthen through your body than it is to stretch as far as possible to the side. Make sure you do not compress the side of your body that you are leaning toward. You should also keep the shoulder of your raised arm back slightly to help open the front of your body.

As you stretch to the side in this pose, you should try to keep both hips on the floor. If one hip lifts off the floor as you move into the stretch, try to encourage your hip to move back down to the floor.

If you want to warm up the sides of your body before holding the pose, you can stretch to the side as described below three times and then hold the pose.

Use caution performing this pose if you have problems with your knees, hips or shoulders.

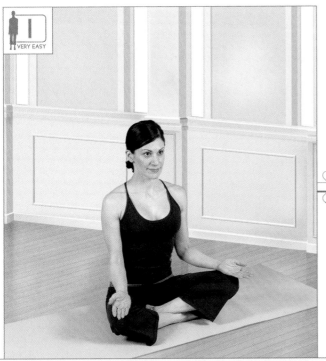

VERY EASY

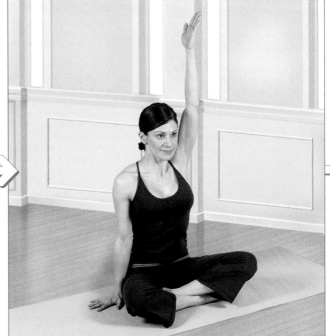

1 Begin in Easy Pose. For information on Easy Pose, see page 74.

2 Relax your shoulders down and back as you lift and expand your chest.

3 Place your right palm on the floor beside your right hip with your fingers pointing to the side.

4 Inhale as you raise your left arm overhead with your palm facing in.

My knees are uncomfortable in this pose. What can I do?

If you have discomfort in your knees or if your hips are stiff, you can sit on the edge of one or two folded blankets. This modification allows you to sit more comfortably and reduces strain on your hips and knees as you perform this pose.

How can I relieve the pressure on my feet in this pose?

If your feet are sore, you can place a folded towel or blanket under your feet to help relieve the pressure.

What can I do if I'm not comfortable sitting on the floor?

You can perform this pose while sitting in an armless chair. Rest one hand in your lap as you stretch your other arm overhead and to the side, as described in the steps below.

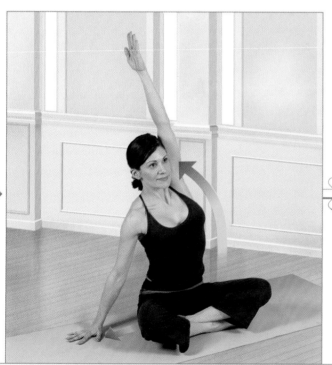

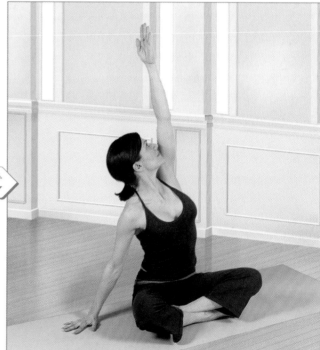

5 Exhale as you stretch to the right, allowing your right hand to slide to the right along the floor.

6 Press both sitting bones toward the floor and extend through the crown of your head to lengthen your spine.

7 Feel the left side of your body lengthening from your hip to your fingertips.

8 Turn your head to look past your left elbow.

9 Hold the pose for 5 to 30 seconds.

10 To come out of the pose, inhale and lift your torso and left arm upright. Then exhale and lower your left arm to return to Easy Pose.

11 Repeat steps 2 to 10 for your other side.

simple twist *(parsva sukhasana)*

Simple Twist helps to increase the flexibility of your spine and upper back. This pose is also useful for stretching your shoulders and upper chest. Performing this pose also massages your abdominal organs, which helps to improve digestion. Simple Twist is commonly used as a warm-up pose and as a counter pose after forward bends and back bends.

As you perform Simple Twist, make sure you keep your hips even and your sitting bones in contact with the floor throughout the pose. Allow the twist to come from your spine, not from your hips.

If you have difficulty sitting with your legs crossed in Simple Twist, you can modify the pose so that one leg is bent and the other leg is extended in front of you. Make sure you twist toward your bent knee and alternate which leg is straight when you switch sides.

You should avoid Simple Twist if you have problems with the discs in your back.

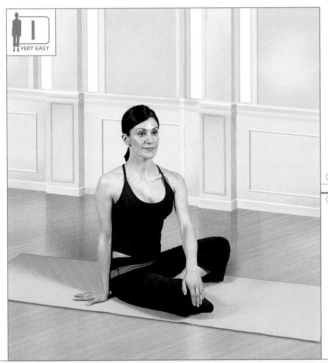
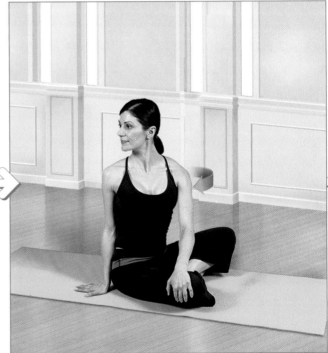

1 Begin in Easy Pose. For information on Easy Pose, see page 74.

2 Turn your upper body toward the right.

3 Place your right palm on the floor behind your right hip, with your fingers pointing behind you.

4 Rest your left palm on your right knee.

5 Exhale as you twist your upper body further to the right.

 • Make sure your sitting bones remain on the floor throughout the pose.

6 Turn your head to look over your right shoulder.

 • If you feel strain in your neck, bring your head back to a neutral position.

How can I modify Simple Twist to open my chest more?

Perform the pose as described in the steps below, except place your hands on top of your shoulders. Your fingers should be on the front your shoulders with your thumbs on the back of your shoulders. As you twist, keep your upper arms parallel to the floor.

What can I do to move deeper into the twist?

To warm up your body and move deeper into the twist, you can twist and release your upper body several times before you hold the pose.

What should I do if I cannot sit straight in Simple Twist?

Try sitting on the edge of two or three thickly folded blankets. This allows your knees to drop so you can sit straight more easily.

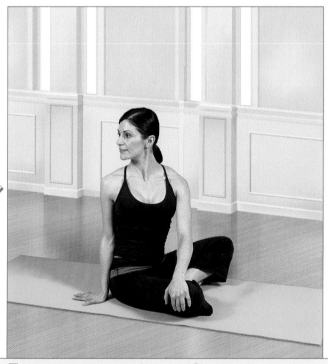

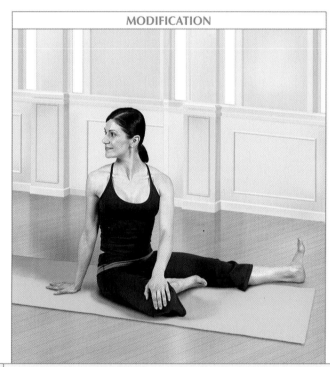

MODIFICATION

7 Point the crown of your head toward the ceiling to lengthen your spine.

• Visualize the twist beginning at the base of your spine, moving up through your spine and continuing through your neck.

8 Hold the pose for 30 seconds to 1 minute. Then return to Easy Pose.

9 Repeat steps 2 to 8 for your other side.

• If you have difficulty sitting in Simple Twist, you can perform the pose with one leg extended in front of you.

1 Begin in Staff Pose. For information on Staff Pose, see page 72.

2 Bend your right leg and place the sole of your right foot against the inside of your left leg. Let your right knee drop toward the floor and then perform the twist. Then repeat for your other side.

seated half
spinal twist *(ardha matsyendrasana)*

Seated Half Spinal Twist is a stimulating pose that helps to increase the flexibility of your spine. You can also use this pose to relieve headaches or stiffness in your neck and shoulders. Performing this pose also massages your abdominal organs, which helps to improve digestion.

As you perform Seated Half Spinal Twist, make sure you keep your hips even and your sitting bones in contact with the floor throughout the pose. Do not allow the twist in this pose to come from your hips.

Instead, you should feel the twist move from the base of your spine up to your neck. Make sure you do not strain your neck trying to look over your shoulder.

If your hips are stiff, you can perform Seated Half Spinal Twist sitting on a folded blanket. This modification supports your pelvis and hips, allowing you to focus on the twist in your spine rather than the position of your hips.

Use caution performing this pose if you have a knee, hip, back or shoulder injury.

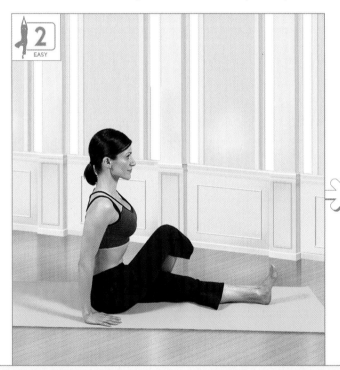
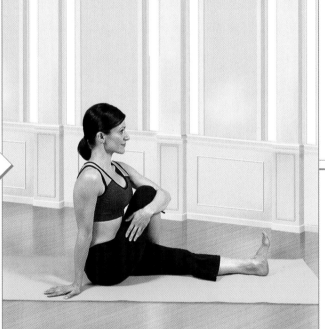

1 Begin in Staff Pose. For information on Staff Pose, see page 72.

2 Bend your right knee and place your right foot on the floor outside your left thigh as close to your hip as is comfortable for you.

• Your knee should point toward the ceiling.

3 Press your sitting bones into the floor and point the crown of your head toward the ceiling.

4 Place your right hand on the floor behind you, close to your body. Your fingers should point behind you.

5 Wrap your left arm around your right knee and then hug your thigh to your torso.

How can I make Seated Half Spinal Twist more challenging for my upper body?

If you are comfortable performing this pose, you can further challenge your upper body by clasping your ankle. Perform steps 1 to 4 below and then move your left elbow to the outside of your right leg. Press your elbow against your thigh to turn your body further to the right. Then clasp your right ankle with your left hand.

How can I make Seated Half Spinal Twist more challenging for my lower body?

If you are comfortable performing this pose, you can further challenge your lower body by bending both knees. Perform steps 1 and 2 below and then bend your left knee and bring your left foot as close to your right hip as possible. Make sure you keep both of your sitting bones on the floor as you perform this modification.

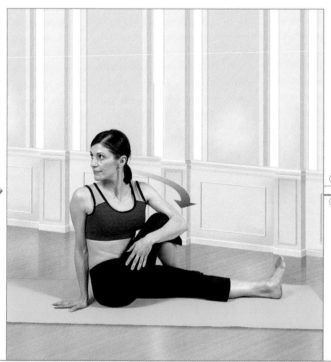

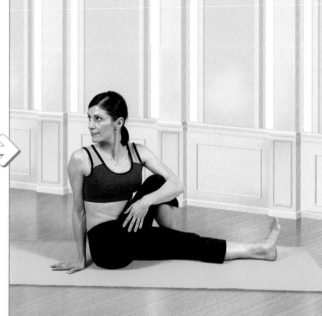

6 Exhale and turn your body to the right.

7 Turn your head to look over your right shoulder.

• If you feel strain in your neck, bring your head back to a neutral position.

8 Press your sitting bones into the floor and point the crown of your head toward the ceiling.

• Make sure your chest is lifted and your shoulders are relaxed and parallel to the floor.

9 Hold the pose for 30 seconds to 1 minute.

10 Repeat steps 1 to 9 for your other side.

seated boat pose *(navasana)*

Seated Boat Pose strengthens your abdominals, lower back and hips, while stretching the back of your legs. Strengthening your abdominal muscles can help protect your lower back and spine. This pose is also beneficial for improving your balance.

In Seated Boat Pose, your legs should be together or only slightly apart. Try to keep your back flat and your spine straight as you straighten your legs. Do not round your lower back or cave in your chest to keep your legs straight. You should also focus on keeping your shoulders back and down. To ensure you are in the correct position, visualize your body forming a V shape.

Use caution performing Seated Boat Pose if you have injured your abdominals, hips or tailbone. Since this is a stimulating pose, you may want to avoid the pose if you have a heart condition or insomnia.

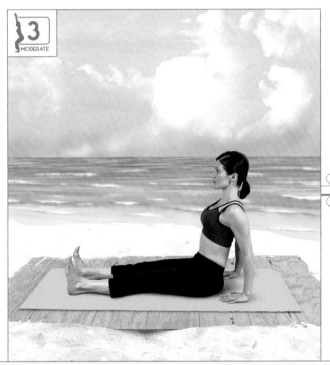
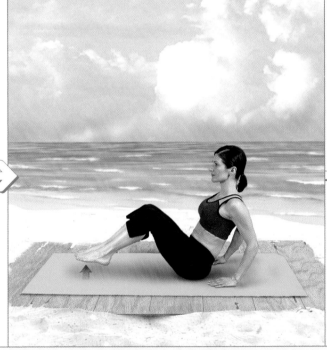

3
MODERATE

1 Begin in Staff Pose. For information on Staff Pose, see page 72.

2 Place your hands on the floor slightly behind your hips, fingers pointing toward your feet.

3 Lift your chest toward the ceiling as you lean back slightly. Make sure your back remains flat.

4 Bend your knees and place your feet together, flat on the floor. Your thighs should be at a 45-degree angle with the floor.

5 Lift your feet one or two inches off the floor, keeping your feet together or slightly apart.

6 Balance on your tailbone and hips.

How can I make Seated Boat Pose easier?

To make the pose easier, bend your knees so that your shins are parallel to the floor. You can also try moving into the pose by straightening one leg at a time.

How can I stretch my inner thighs in Seated Boat Pose?

Perform the pose as described below, except separate your legs until they form a V shape. Make sure you can maintain your balance and keep your back flat as you separate your legs.

Can I use a strap to help straighten my legs in Seated Boat Pose?

Yes. With your knees bent, loop a strap around the soles of your feet and grip an end of the strap in each hand. Inhale and lean your torso back and then straighten your legs as you push your feet against the strap. Keep the strap taut, but do not pull on the strap.

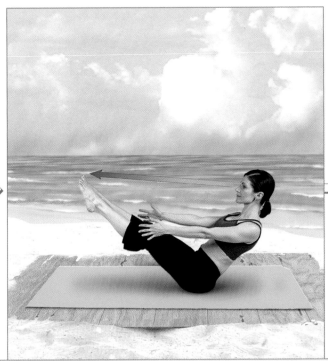

7 Inhale and slowly straighten your legs until the tips of your toes are slightly above your eye level.

8 Bring your arms forward at shoulder height, parallel to the floor with your palms facing in.

9 Relax your shoulders down away from your ears.

• If you cannot keep your balance, you can leave your hands on the floor behind your hips.

10 Tip your chin slightly toward your chest to lengthen the back of your neck.

11 Hold the pose for 10 seconds to 1 minute and then exhale as you lower your legs to the floor. Then return to Staff Pose.

• After performing Seated Boat Pose, you should perform Seated Forward Bend to relieve your lower back. For information on Seated Forward Bend, see page 100.

thunderbolt pose *(vajrasana)*

Thunderbolt Pose is a simple seated pose that stretches your thighs, knees, ankles and feet. This pose also helps improve your seated posture. Thunderbolt Pose is considered one of the safer seated poses for people with back problems.

You may find this pose useful for meditation because you can easily keep your spine straight and your upper body relaxed. Thunderbolt Pose is a great alternative to Lotus Pose for meditation, especially if you find Lotus Pose too intense.

You can place a folded blanket under your hips if your knees feel strained or you find it difficult to sit on your heels due to tightness in your thighs. If you find kneeling on the floor uncomfortable, you can kneel on a folded blanket to pad your knees, shins and the top of your feet. Only remain in the pose for as long as you feel comfortable.

Make sure you avoid the pose if you have an injury to your knees or ankles.

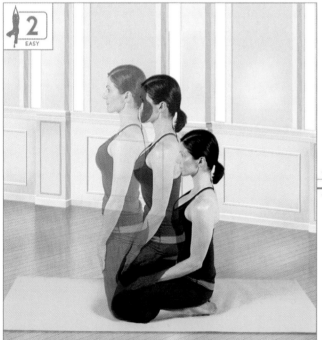
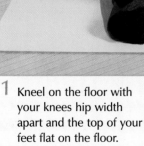

1 Kneel on the floor with your knees hip width apart and the top of your feet flat on the floor.

2 Exhale as you sit back onto your heels.

3 Place your hands on top of your thighs close to your knees, with your palms facing down.

4 Relax your shoulders and upper body, but keep your spine straight and tall.

5 Point the crown of your head toward the ceiling and gaze straight ahead.

6 Hold the pose for 30 seconds to 1 minute.

• After performing Thunderbolt Pose, you should shake out your legs to help relieve your knees, ankles and feet.

How can I stretch my feet more in Thunderbolt Pose?

Perform the pose as described in the steps below, except curl your toes under to rest the balls of your feet on the floor.

How can I even out the pressure on my feet in this pose?

You may feel more pressure on the inner top of your feet in this pose. To even out the pressure between the inner and outer top of your feet, gently press the outer edges of your feet toward the floor.

How can I modify Thunderbolt Pose to help relieve tension in my face?

You can perform Lion Pose to stretch your face and neck as you perform Thunderbolt Pose. To perform Lion Pose, open your mouth wide and stick your tongue out toward your chin and then exhale as you say "Haaaa." You should be careful performing Lion Pose if you have an injury to your face, neck or tongue.

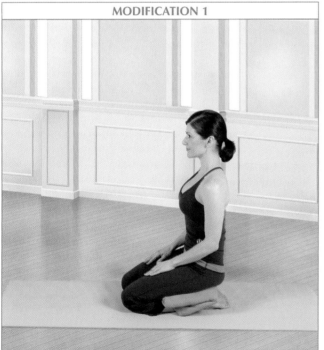

| MODIFICATION 1 | MODIFICATION 2 |

1 If you feel any discomfort in your knees or you cannot sit on your heels, place a cushion or folded blanket between your hips and heels.

• You can stretch your arms and hands while performing Thunderbolt Pose.

1 Perform Thunderbolt Pose, except raise both arms to shoulder height in front of you.

2 Interlace your fingers and rotate your wrists so your palms face forward. Inhale as you raise your arms to face your palms toward the ceiling.

hero pose *(virasana)*

Hero Pose increases the flexibility of your legs by providing a deep stretch to your knees, ankles and the top of your thighs and feet. This pose is often used in breathing practices and meditation. The name of the pose comes from the Sanskrit word *vira*, which means hero or warrior.

When you first start practicing Hero Pose, you may find that you cannot sit on the floor between your feet. If you cannot sit on the floor, you can sit on a prop,

such as a block or folded blanket. You can gradually lower the height of the prop when you feel less pressure on your knees and a less intense stretch in your thighs. It may take several weeks of practice before you can sit on the floor between your feet. Never strain your knees in an attempt to sit on the floor.

You should avoid performing Hero Pose if you have a knee or ankle injury.

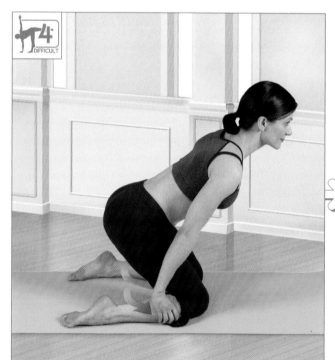

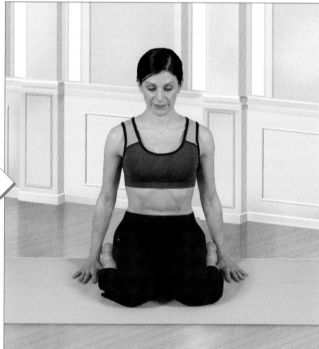

1 Kneel on the floor with your knees hip width apart and your thighs parallel.

2 Move your feet a little more than hip width apart, keeping the top of your feet flat on the floor.

3 Lean forward and then use your hands to turn the fleshy part of your calves outward.

4 Exhale as you sit on the floor between your feet.

• If you feel any discomfort in your knees or you cannot sit on the floor, place a prop, such as a block, thick book or folded blanket, between your feet and sit on the prop.

How can I stretch my upper body in Hero Pose?

Interlace your fingers and then extend your arms forward, parallel to the floor. Turn your palms away from your torso so your thumbs are pointing toward the floor. Inhale as you raise your arms above your head until your palms are facing the ceiling. Be sure to keep your neck long and your shoulders relaxed. Stretching your upper body in Hero Pose can help reduce stiffness in your neck and shoulders and open your chest, increasing your ability to take deeper breaths.

The top of my feet hurt when I perform Hero Pose. What can I do?

If the top of your feet hurt while performing Hero Pose, you can place a folded towel or blanket under your feet. Placing a folded towel or blanket under your feet can also help reduce any strain you may be experiencing in your knees.

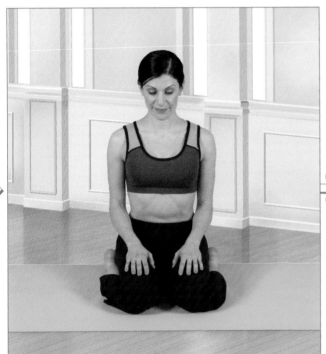

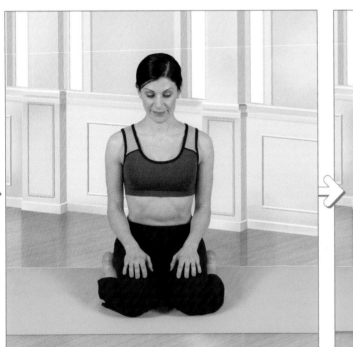

5 Place your hands on the top of your thighs close to your knees, with your palms facing down.

6 Relax your shoulders and upper body, keeping your spine straight and tall.

7 Point the crown of your head toward the ceiling and gaze straight ahead.

• Visualize yourself as a warrior sitting tall and proud.

8 Hold the pose for 30 seconds to 1 minute.

• After performing Hero Pose, you should shake out your legs to help relieve your knees, ankles and feet.

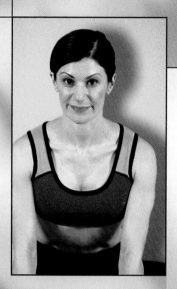

Chapter 5

Seated forward bends are good for stretching your lower back and often your hamstrings. You may also find that seated forward bends produce a calming effect on your body and mind. Seated forward bends are especially beneficial when performed after back bends, twists and side bends because forward bends release your lower back and return your spine to a neutral position. In this chapter, you will learn how to perform a number of seated forward bends.

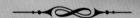

Seated Forward Bends

In this Chapter...

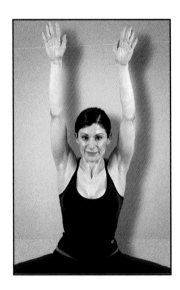

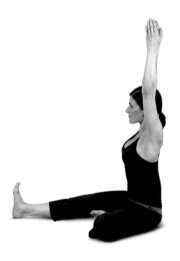

easy pose
forward bend

Easy Pose Forward Bend provides a good stretch to your groin and inner thighs, while strengthening your back. This pose also develops flexibility in your hips and knees, as well as stimulating your abdominal organs, which can help aid digestion. Performing this pose can also soothe your nervous system, which helps clear and calm your mind.

As you bend forward in this pose, you should focus on lowering your abdomen and chest, rather than your forehead. Keep in mind that lengthening your spine is more important than trying to bend forward as far as

possible. After performing Easy Pose Forward Bend, you should shake out your legs to help relieve your knees and ankles.

If your hips are stiff or your knees feel strained in this pose, sitting on thickly folded blankets may make the pose more comfortable. Sitting on blankets can also help prevent your lower back from rounding.

Make sure you use caution performing this pose if you have problems with your knees, hips, lower back or spine.

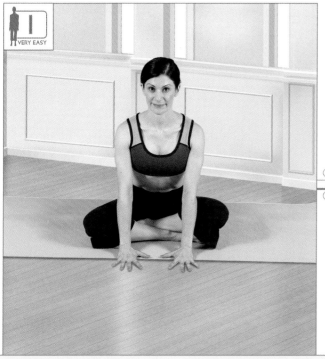

VERY EASY

1 Begin in Easy Pose. For information on Easy Pose, see page 74.

2 Press your sitting bones into the floor and point the crown of your head toward the ceiling to lengthen your spine.

3 Place your palms on the floor in front of you.

4 Spread your fingers out, with your middle fingers pointing forward.

5 Exhale as you bend forward from your hips and slide your hands forward along the floor.

6 Keep your back straight as long as possible and then relax your shoulders and head forward.

7 Hold the pose for 15 to 30 seconds and then inhale as you slowly curl up to return to Easy Pose.

8 Repeat steps 1 to 7 placing the opposite leg on top in step 1.

bound angle forward bend

Bound Angle Forward Bend provides a great stretch to your groin and inner thighs, while strengthening your back. This pose also stimulates your abdominals and helps to develop flexibility in your hips, knees, ankles and feet.

If you are feeling anxious, fatigued or mildly depressed, you can perform this pose to help soothe your nervous system and clear your mind.

You should focus on lowering your abdomen and chest, rather than your forehead, as you bend forward in this pose. Keep in mind that maintaining length in

your spine is more important than trying to bend forward as far as possible.

Allow your knees to drop toward the floor in this pose, but make sure you do not force your knees down. If your knees are high up off the floor, move your feet further away from your groin or place rolled up blankets under your knees for support.

Use caution performing Bound Angle Forward Bend if you have problems with your spine, lower back, hips, groin or knees.

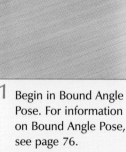

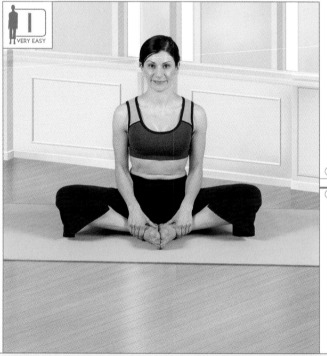

1 Begin in Bound Angle Pose. For information on Bound Angle Pose, see page 76.

2 Press your sitting bones into the floor and point the crown of your head toward the ceiling to lengthen your spine.

3 Clasp your ankles or toes with your hands.

4 Exhale as you bend forward from your hips.

5 As you bend forward, keep your back straight as long as possible and then relax your shoulders and head forward.

• Allow your forearms to move in front of your shins.

6 Hold the pose for 15 to 30 seconds and then inhale as you slowly curl up to return to Bound Angle Pose.

head to knee pose *(janu sirsasana)*

Head to Knee Pose provides an intense stretch to the back of your legs, particularly your straight leg. This pose also stretches the back of your waist and lengthens your spine.

Although this pose is called Head to Knee Pose, you should focus on lowering your abdomen toward your thigh instead of trying to reach your head down to your knee. You should also focus on keeping your sitting bones in even contact with the floor as you drop your bent knee toward the floor. If your bent

knee is high up off the floor, you can move your foot further away from your groin.

When you first start practicing this pose, you may find you cannot bend very far forward. Keep in mind that maintaining a straight and lengthened spine is more important than bending forward as far as possible. If necessary, you can use a strap around the foot of your straight leg for support as you bend forward.

Avoid performing this pose if you have slipped discs in your back or knee or back problems.

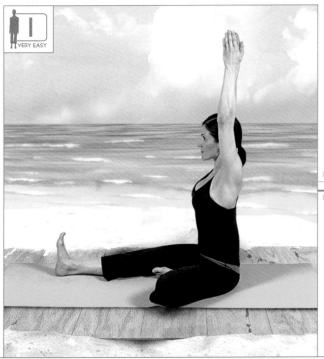

VERY EASY

1 Begin in Staff Pose. For information on Staff Pose, see page 72.

2 Bend your left leg and place the sole of your left foot against the inside of your right thigh. Let your left knee drop toward the floor.

• Your right foot should be flexed, with your toes pointing toward the ceiling.

3 Inhale as you raise your arms above your head, with your palms facing each other.

4 Exhale as you bend forward from your hips over your right leg. Then clasp the sides of your right leg or foot.

5 Drop your pelvis forward and down to lengthen your spine.

• Keep your head, neck and spine in a straight line.

6 Press forward through the heel of your right foot and the crown of your head as you press back through your sitting bones.

How can I make Head to Knee Pose easier?

You can place your palms on the floor on either side of your straight leg. This modification reduces the strain in the back of your straight leg and also helps keep your head, neck and spine in a straight line as you bend forward. If you still feel a lot of tension or discomfort in the back of your straight leg, you can bend the knee of your straight leg slightly. As you gain more flexibility, straighten your leg a little more each time you perform the pose.

How can I prevent my lower back from rounding in Head to Knee Pose?

Sitting on a cushion or folded blankets can help prevent your lower back from rounding in this pose. This modification also supports your pelvis and helps to relieve tension in your lower back and the back of your straight leg.

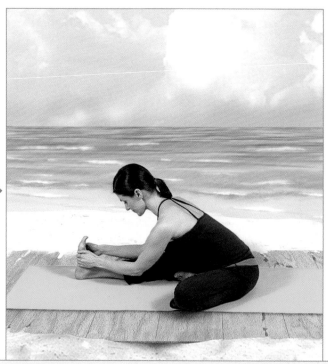

MODIFICATION

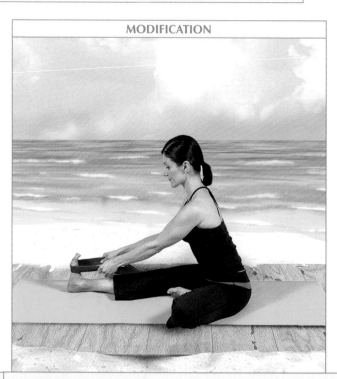

7 Hold the pose for 15 to 30 seconds, releasing further into the pose with each exhalation. Then return to Staff Pose.

8 Repeat steps 2 to 7 with your right leg bent.

• After performing Head to Knee Pose, perform Inclined Plane Pose as a counter pose. See page 212.

• You can perform Head to Knee Pose using a strap for support.

1 Perform Head to Knee Pose, except wrap a strap around the foot of your straight leg and hold an end of the strap in each hand.

• Make sure you do not use the strap to pull yourself forward.

seated forward
bend *(paschimottanasana)*

Seated Forward Bend provides an intense stretch to the back of your body, especially to your spine and the back of your legs. This pose can help rejuvenate your body when you are tired or ill.

When you first start practicing this pose, you may not be able to bend very far forward due to tightness in your hamstrings. Make sure you do not force your upper body forward. Instead, try sitting on the edge of a thickly folded blanket, which can relieve tension in the back of your legs. Sitting on a blanket also

supports your pelvis and helps keep your spine straight and lengthened.

As you bend forward, you should focus on lowering your abdomen and your chest, rather than your forehead. Keep in mind that lengthening your spine is more important than trying to bend forward as far as possible. Try to release your body further into the pose with each exhalation.

Avoid performing this pose if you have lower back problems or slipped discs in your back.

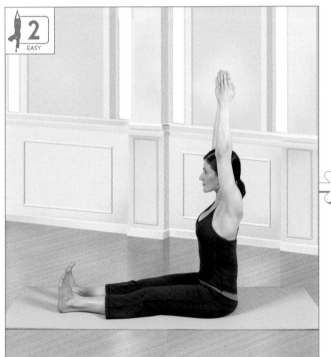

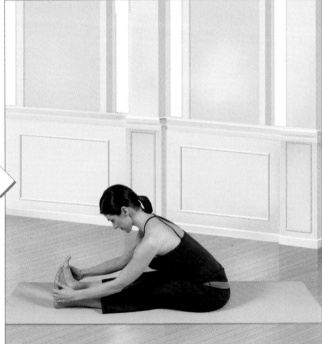

1 Begin in Staff Pose. For information on Staff Pose, see page 72.

- Your feet should be flexed, with your toes pointing toward the ceiling.

2 Inhale as you raise your arms above your head and lengthen your spine. Your palms should be shoulder width apart and facing each other.

- Your shoulders should be relaxed.

3 Exhale as you bend forward from your hips and stretch your hands toward your feet. Then clasp the sides of your legs or feet.

4 Drop your pelvis forward and down to further lengthen your spine, keeping your neck and shoulders relaxed.

- Keep your head, neck and spine in a straight line.

My legs feel tight while performing Seated Forward Bend. What should I do?

If you experience tension or discomfort in the back of your legs while in the pose, keep your legs slightly bent to reduce the tension. When your knees are bent, you can support your upper body by placing your palms on the floor on either side of your legs. As you gain flexibility, straighten your legs a little more each time you perform the pose.

Is there another way to release further into the pose?

Before holding the pose, raise and lower your upper body two or three times, stretching a little further forward each time you bend forward. This movement is especially useful for beginners.

I cannot bend very far forward in this pose. What can I do?

If you cannot bend very far forward, you may want to use a bolster to support your upper body. This allows you to focus more on relaxing your upper body forward.

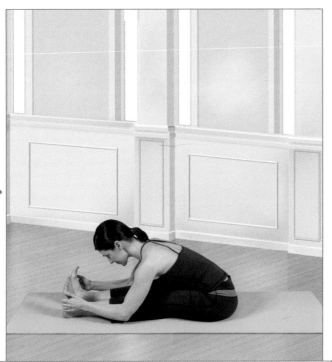

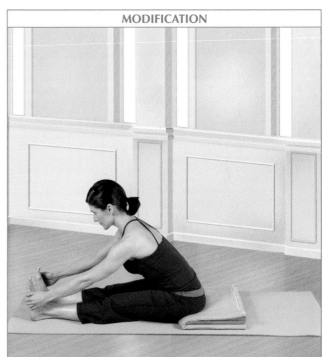

MODIFICATION

5 Press forward through your heels and the crown of your head as you press back through your sitting bones.

6 Hold the pose for 15 to 30 seconds. Then return to Staff Pose.

• After performing Seated Forward Bend, perform Inclined Plane Pose as a counter pose. See page 212.

1 Perform Seated Forward Bend sitting on the edge of a thickly folded blanket.

• Sitting on a blanket relieves tension in the back of your legs, supports your pelvis and helps keep your spine straight and lengthened while you are in the pose.

seated wide angle
forward bend *(upavista konasana)*

Seated Wide Angle Forward Bend provides a stretch to your inner thighs and hamstrings. This pose can also help calm your mind and relieve stress.

As you bend forward in this pose, you may be tempted to round your back. To prevent rounding your back, make sure you bend forward from your hips and lean forward with your chest, not your forehead. Lengthening your spine is more important than trying to bend forward as far as possible.

In this pose, make sure your legs never form an angle greater than 90 degrees, which may strain the ligaments in your hips. You should also make sure your knees are not locked. As you hold the pose, visualize your body softening with each exhalation.

This pose is easier on your ankles and knees than some other seated poses, such Hero Pose or Easy Pose. However, you should use caution performing this pose if you have a knee or hip injury.

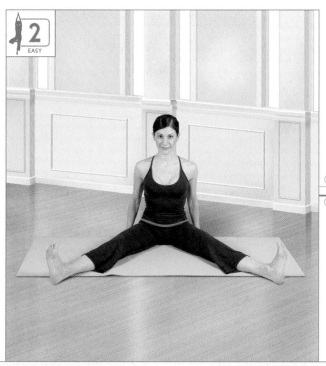

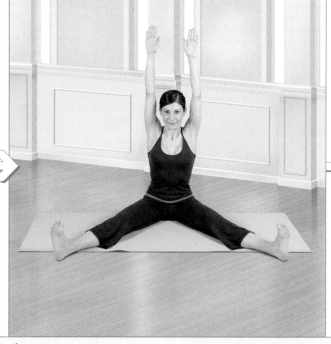

1 Begin in Staff Pose. For information on Staff Pose, see page 72.

2 Keep your spine straight as you spread your legs as far apart as is comfortable for you.

• Make sure your legs are straight, with your knees and toes pointing toward the ceiling.

3 Press the back of your thighs firmly into the floor.

4 Inhale as you raise your arms overhead, with your palms shoulder width apart and facing forward.

• Your elbows should be straight but not locked. Your shoulders should be relaxed.

My legs feel tight while performing Seated Wide Angle Forward Bend. What should I do?

If you experience tightness in your inner thighs or hamstrings while in the pose, do not try to force yourself to the floor. Instead, sit on the edge of a folded blanket and rest your upper body on a bolster or chair. This can help reduce the strain in your legs and is also useful for modifying the pose if you have back problems.

Can I bend my knees while performing Seated Wide Angle Forward Bend?

If you have a lot of difficulty bending forward, you can bend your knees slightly in order to bend forward. As you bend forward with your knees slightly bent, make sure your kneecaps are pointing toward the ceiling.

Can I perform Seated Wide Angle Forward Bend if I have a stiff back?

Yes. You can sit with your back against a wall, but do not bend your upper body forward. This allows you to stretch your legs in the pose without straining your back.

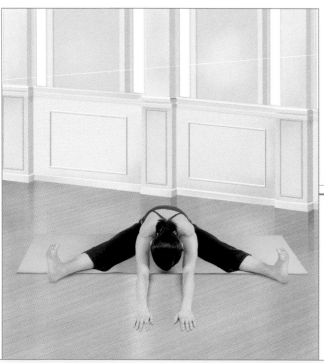

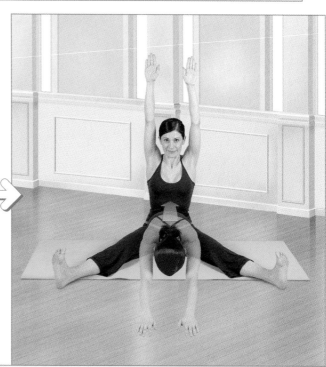

5 Keeping your arms straight, exhale as you bend forward from your hips and place your palms on the floor between your legs.

• Your back should be straight and flat.

6 Release your pelvis forward and down to lengthen your spine.

• Make sure you keep your head, neck and shoulders relaxed and in a straight line.

7 Hold the pose for 15 seconds to 1 minute.

8 To come out of the pose, inhale as you lift your arms and upper body toward the ceiling to return to a seated position. Then exhale as you bring your arms back to your sides. Return to Staff Pose.

seated yoga
mudra pose *(yoga mudra)*

Seated Yoga Mudra Pose, also known as The Seal of Yoga, provides an intense stretch for your shoulders and upper back, which may help to relieve tightness in these areas. This pose also stretches your neck and stimulates your abdominal area. You may find that this pose not only clears your mind, but also reconnects your heart and mind to help you become more aware of your feelings.

As you bend forward in this pose, your buttocks may lift off your heels slightly. With practice, you should be able to keep your buttocks on your heels as you perform the pose. You should also try to keep your palms together to maintain the intensity of the stretch in your shoulders. Stretching your arms back and up can help improve circulation in your hands and also help correct a rounded back and shoulders.

After performing the pose, you should shake out your legs to relieve your knees, ankles and feet.

Use caution performing Seated Yoga Mudra Pose if you have neck, shoulder, arm or knee problems.

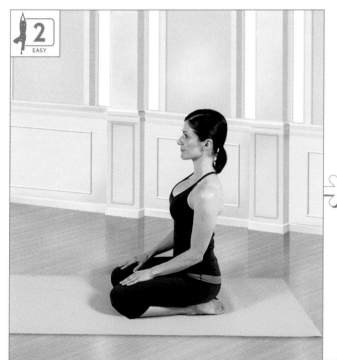
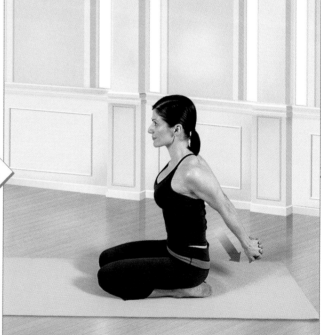

1 Kneel on the floor with your knees hip width apart and the top of your feet flat on the floor.

2 Exhale as you sit back onto your heels.

3 Place your hands on top of your thighs close to your knees, with your palms facing down.

4 Relax your shoulders and upper body, keeping your spine straight and tall.

5 Interlace your fingers behind your back.

6 Inhale as you press your hands down away from your shoulders to lengthen your arms.

• Feel your shoulder blades come together as your chest opens.

I have difficulty interlacing my fingers behind my back. What can I do?

You can hold a strap with your hands as close together as is comfortable for you. This modification places less strain on your shoulders.

What should I do if my forehead does not reach the floor in this pose?

If you have difficulty reaching your forehead to the floor, you can place a folded blanket on the floor in front of you to support your head.

I cannot sit back onto my heels in Seated Yoga Mudra Pose. What can I do?

If you cannot sit back onto your heels, you can place a thickly folded blanket between your heels and buttocks and sit on the blanket. Sitting on a folded blanket can also help reduce any strain you may be experiencing in your knees and hips.

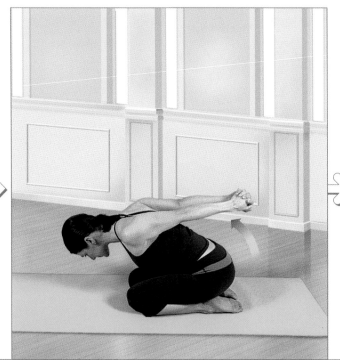

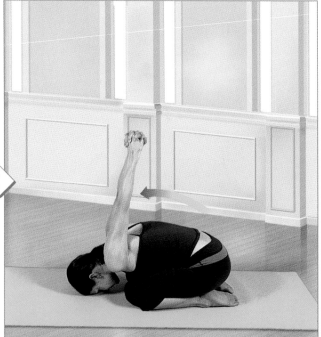

7 Exhale as you bend forward from your hips.

8 Inhale as you raise your arms behind you as far as is comfortable for you.

• Your forehead moves further toward the floor as your arms move away from your body.

9 Continue to lift your hands and lower your forehead toward the floor.

10 Hold the pose for 30 seconds to 1 minute.

11 To come out of the pose, press out through your hands and keep your back flat as you inhale and lift your torso up.

child's pose *(balasana)*

Child's Pose is a seated forward bend that stretches and releases your spine and lower back. You can use this pose as a warm-up pose, a resting pose or a counter pose after performing a back bend.

While performing Child's Pose, you should feel your spine lengthen as you drop the weight of your hips toward your heels and relax your head to the floor. Make sure you do not rest your weight on your neck and forehead. You should also breathe evenly while performing the pose and visualize your body softening with each breath.

To stretch your shoulders in this pose, you can extend your arms forward, instead of placing them by your sides. If your forehead does not reach the floor or if you feel too much pressure on your forehead in this pose, you can rest your forehead on your folded arms.

Child's Pose is a simple pose that is comfortable and safe for almost everyone. However, you should avoid this pose if you have knee problems or high blood pressure.

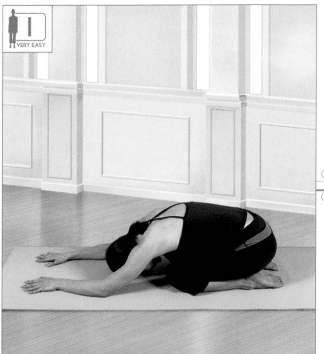

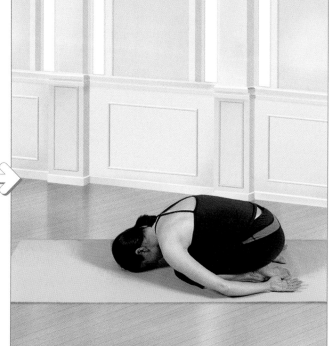

VERY EASY

1 Begin in Table Pose. For information on Table Pose, see page 172.

2 Maintaining the position of your hands, exhale as you sit back onto your heels and lay your upper body on your thighs.

3 Rest your forehead on the floor.

4 Place your arms by your sides, with your hands by your feet and your palms facing up.

5 Exhale as you release your hips toward your heels and feel your spine lengthening.

6 Hold the pose for 15 seconds to 2 minutes.

7 To come out of the pose, inhale as you press your hands into the floor to lift yourself to a seated position.

Can I modify Child's Pose to make the pose more relaxing?

Yes. You can use a bolster to make this pose more relaxing and restorative. Move your knees wider than hip width apart and place a bolster between your knees. You can then rest your upper body, arms and head on the bolster. This modification is also useful if you are pregnant or very overweight.

I cannot sit back onto my heels in Child's Pose. What can I do?

If you cannot sit back onto your heels in this pose, you can place a thickly folded blanket between your heels and buttocks and sit on the blanket. Sitting on a folded blanket can also help reduce any strain you may be experiencing in your knees and hips. If you still find Child's Pose uncomfortable, you can perform Little Boat Pose instead. For information on Little Boat Pose, see page 58.

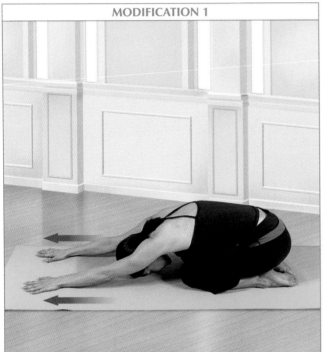

MODIFICATION 1

- You can perform Child's Pose with your arms extended. This modification is known as Extended Child's Pose and stretches your shoulders, back and hips.

1 Perform Child's Pose, except leave your arms extended and relax your shoulders and arms toward the floor.

MODIFICATION 2

- You can perform Child's Pose with your forehead resting on your arms. This is useful if your forehead does not reach the floor or you feel too much pressure on your forehead while performing the pose.

1 Perform Child's Pose, except fold your arms in front of you and rest your forehead on your arms.

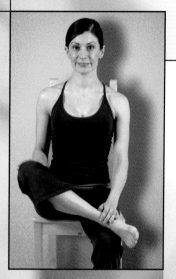

Chapter 6

Chair Poses are a great alternative to seated poses if you have difficulty sitting on the floor and cannot perform seated poses easily. For this reason, chair poses are ideal for seniors and people with limited mobility. You may also find chair poses useful if you want to fit in a yoga practice while sitting at your desk at work. You can perform the chair poses in this chapter to help release tension and increase flexibility in your body.

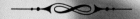

Chair Poses

In this Chapter...

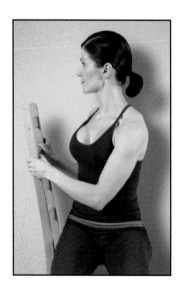

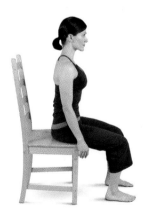

seated mountain pose

Seated Mountain Pose helps you focus on your seated posture and improve the alignment of your spine. When your body is aligned correctly, your head, neck and spine form a straight line. This pose also serves as a starting position for many other chair poses.

Seated Mountain Pose is a calming pose that allows you to develop an awareness of your breath, which is ideal for meditation. You may also find that this pose helps you feel mentally grounded and stable.

While performing Seated Mountain Pose, your lower body from your waist down should feel stable and grounded, while your upper body should feel light and relaxed. To help achieve this feeling, visualize your head and torso rising away from your legs and feet.

If your feet do not reach the floor in this pose, you can place a prop, such as a stack of books, under your feet. When resting your feet on a prop, make sure your knees are not higher than your hips and your thighs are parallel to the floor.

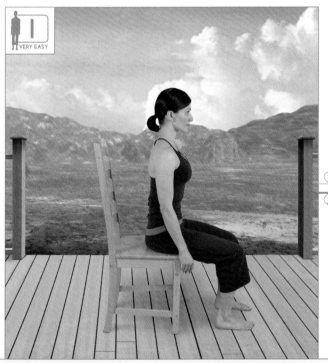

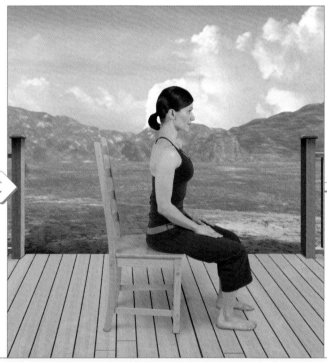

1 Sit upright on the front half of a chair.

- Make sure you do not lean back into the chair.

2 Place your feet on the floor, with your knees and feet hip width apart and your toes pointing forward.

- Make sure your thighs are parallel to the floor and your knees are no higher than your hips.

3 Rest your palms on your thighs.

4 Press your sitting bones into the seat of the chair.

- Your lower body should feel fully supported by the chair seat and the floor.

Is there another way to stretch my arms and shoulders in this pose?

Yes. You can interlace your fingers and turn your wrists so your palms face outward. Then inhale as you stretch your arms above your head. As you exhale, press the crown of your head toward the ceiling and relax your shoulder blades down and back. Stretching your arms and shoulders in this way can help reduce stiffness in your neck and shoulders, as well as open your chest.

How can I incorporate movement into Seated Mountain Pose?

Position your hands in Prayer Pose, as shown on page 48. Inhale and lift your arms overhead and then exhale and lower your hands back to chest level. Repeat this movement three to six times before holding the pose.

How can I release tension in my shoulders and upper back in this pose?

Perform the arm position of Eagle Pose by performing steps 2 to 4 on page 146. Repeat these steps crossing your other arm over.

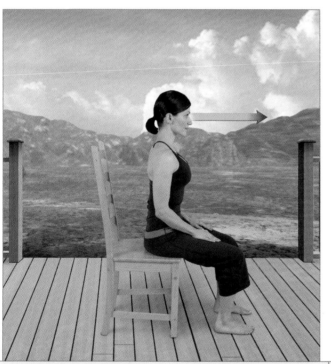

MODIFICATION

5 Point the crown of your head toward the ceiling and gaze straight ahead.

6 Relax your shoulders down and back.

• Visualize your spine lengthening and your rib cage lifting and expanding.

7 Hold the pose for 30 seconds to 1 minute.

• You can perform Seated Mountain Pose with your arms extended over your head. This modification stretches your arms and shoulders.

1 Inhale as you raise your arms above your head, keeping your shoulders relaxed down.

• Your arms should be shoulder width apart and your palms should be facing each other.

2 Hold the pose for 30 seconds to 1 minute.

chair hip stretch

You can perform Chair Hip Stretch to open and stretch your hips. You may find this stretch beneficial after you have been sitting in a chair all day long.

If you have difficulty sitting on the floor, you can practice Chair Hip Stretch to develop the flexibility your hips require to perform seated poses, such as Half Lotus Pose. You can also perform Chair Hip Stretch as an alternative to Bound Angle Pose if you find it difficult to sit on the floor.

While performing this pose, make sure you do not use too much force to press your knee down. You should feel a comfortable stretch in your hip and should not feel any strain.

You should use caution performing Chair Hip Stretch if you have problems with your hips or knees.

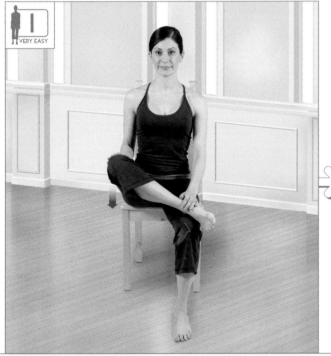
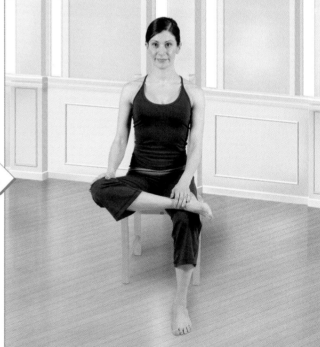

1 Begin in Seated Mountain Pose. For information on Seated Mountain Pose, see page 110.

2 Place your right ankle on top of your left knee.

3 Rest your right hand on your right leg, just above your right knee.

4 Exhale as you gently press your right knee toward the floor.

5 Inhale as you release the press on your knee.

6 Press and release your knee three times and then return to Seated Mountain Pose.

7 Repeat steps 2 to 6 for your other side.

seated knee to chest pose

Seated Knee to Chest Pose stretches your hips and thighs. You can also use this pose to strengthen your back and open your chest. Bringing your knee toward your chest in this pose stimulates your abdominal area, which can help improve digestion and elimination.

If you spend most of the day sitting in a chair at work, you may want to use this pose to take a break and stretch. Like all chair poses, this pose is also a good alternative to seated poses if you do not feel comfortable sitting on the floor.

While performing Seated Knee to Chest Pose, make sure your foot remains flat on the floor as you lift your other leg. Also, remember to keep your shoulders relaxed down throughout the pose.

If you have lower back problems, you can perform the pose without arching your back. Instead, remain sitting up straight as you lift your knee toward your chest. You should also approach this pose with caution if you have problems with your hips.

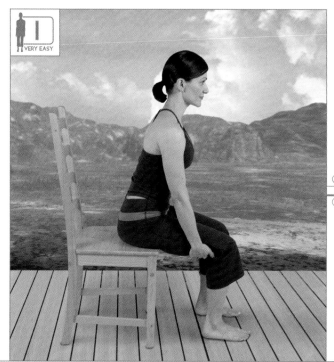
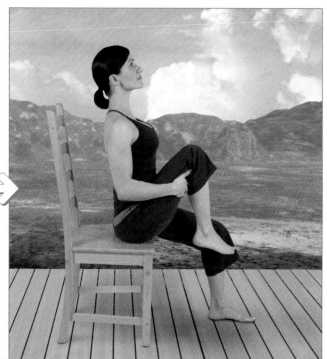

VERY EASY

1 Begin in Seated Mountain Pose. For information on Seated Mountain Pose, see page 110.

2 Interlace your fingers under your right thigh.

3 Press your sitting bones into the seat of the chair and the crown of your head toward the ceiling.

4 Relax your shoulders down.

5 Lift your right knee up toward your chest.

6 Inhale as you arch your back and raise your head to look up at the ceiling.

• Make sure you keep the back of your neck long.

7 Hold the pose for 15 to 30 seconds and then exhale as you return to Seated Mountain Pose.

8 Repeat steps 2 to 7 for your other side.

chair forward bend

You can perform Chair Forward Bend to relieve tension in your head, neck and shoulders. You may also find this pose soothes your nervous system and encourages your mind to let go of stress.

Bending forward in this pose stretches the back of your body and stimulates your abdominal area, which helps to improve digestion. If you are feeling tired or ill, bending forward in this way is helpful for rejuvenating your body. This pose is also useful if you have been sitting in a chair all day at work.

As you bend forward, you should focus on keeping your spine lengthened and lowering your abdomen and chest, rather than your forehead. As you hold the pose, try to release your body further into the pose with each exhalation.

If you find this pose strains your shoulders, you can rest your arms by your sides as you bend forward. You should use caution performing Chair Forward Bend if you have high blood pressure or a headache.

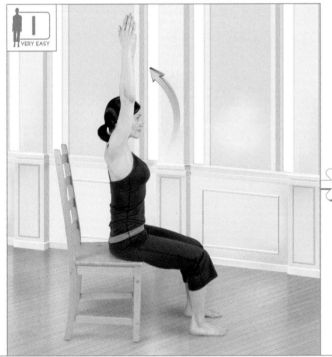

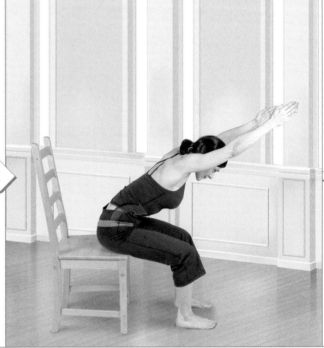

VERY EASY

1 Begin in Seated Mountain Pose. For information on Seated Mountain Pose, see page 110.

2 Inhale as you raise your arms above your head and lengthen your spine. Your palms should be shoulder width apart and facing each other.

• Your shoulders should be relaxed down and back.

3 Exhale as you bend forward from your hips and stretch your hands forward.

• Your upper arms should be beside your ears.

4 Drop your pelvis forward and down to further lengthen your spine.

• Keep your head, neck and spine in a straight line.

How can I modify the pose if I have high blood pressure or a headache?

You can perform a modification that keeps your head above your heart. Perform the pose as described in the steps below, except position your chair close to a table. As you bend forward, rest your forearms on the table. Place each palm on the opposite elbow and rest your head on your forearms. As you exhale, drop your pelvis forward to lengthen your spine and relax your shoulders and arms.

What should I do with my hands in this pose?

You should place your hands in a position that feels comfortable. If your hands reach the floor, you can rest your palms or the back of your hands on the floor. If you rest the back of your hands on the floor, you can place your toes and the balls of your feet on your palms, with your fingers pointing toward your heels, to massage your feet.

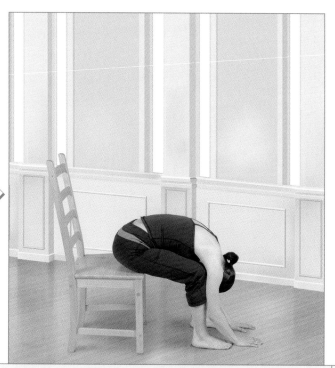

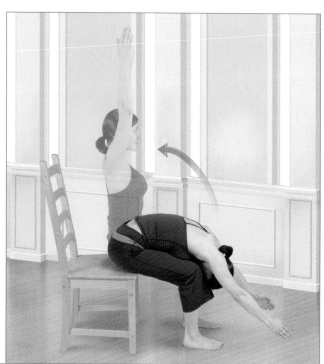

5 Relax your neck and shoulders, allowing your head and arms to hang toward the floor.

6 Hold the pose for 5 seconds to 1 minute, breathing through your entire body and releasing further into the pose with each exhalation.

Come Out of the Pose

1 Bring your upper arms beside your ears.

2 Press your feet into the floor and your sitting bones into the seat of the chair.

3 Inhale and come up to a sitting position, keeping your back flat.

4 Exhale and bring your arms down to your sides.

chair twist

Chair Twist helps to increase the flexibility of your spine and back, while stretching your shoulders and chest. You can perform this pose to relieve stiffness in your neck, shoulders and upper back. Twisting in this pose also massages your abdominal organs, which helps to improve digestion.

When performing the pose, you should use a chair without arms so you can sit sideways on the chair. Make sure your hips are square to the front and your sitting bones remain in contact with the seat of the chair throughout the pose.

As you twist in this pose, do not pull on the back of the chair. Only use the chair for support as you twist your spine. You may find it helpful to visualize the twist beginning at the base of your spine, moving up through your spine and continuing through your neck.

Use caution performing Chair Twist if you have problems with the discs in your back.

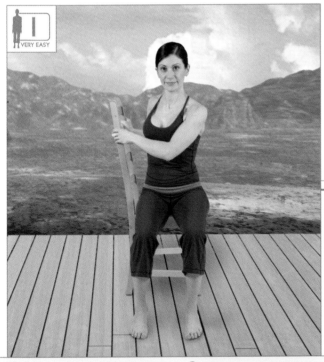

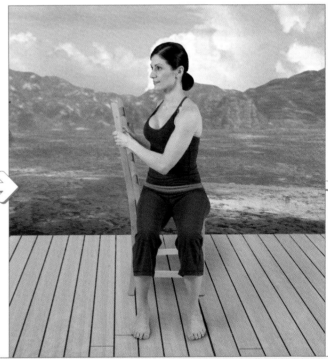

1 Begin in Seated Mountain Pose, with the right side of your body facing the chair back. For information on Seated Mountain Pose, see page 110.

2 Hold the sides of the chair back with your hands at approximately shoulder height.

• Make sure your hips and torso are facing forward and your shoulders are relaxed and down.

3 Inhale as you press your sitting bones into the seat of the chair and the crown of your head toward the ceiling.

4 Exhale and twist to the right from the base of your spine.

What can I do to warm up my body and move deeper into the twist?

On each side, perform the twist three times and then hold the pose.

Can I perform a variation of Chair Twist that stretches the sides of my body?

Yes. Begin in Seated Mountain Pose. Place your left hand on the outside of your right thigh and extend your right arm above your head. Then twist to the right. Repeat this variation for your other side.

Is there another variation of Chair Twist that I can perform?

Yes. Begin in Seated Mountain Pose. Cross your right knee over your left thigh and then place your left hand on the outside of your right knee. Inhale as you lift your chest up to lengthen your spine. Then exhale as you twist your upper body to the right and gaze over your right shoulder. Twist and release your upper body three to five times. Repeat this variation for your other side.

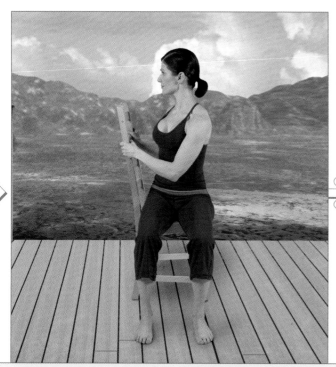

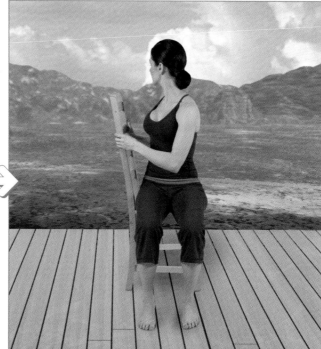

5 Inhale as you press your sitting bones into the seat of the chair and the crown of your head toward the ceiling.

6 Then exhale and twist up through the middle of your spine.

- Make sure you do not pull on the chair back as you twist.

7 Inhale as you press your sitting bones into the seat of the chair and the crown of your head toward the ceiling.

8 Then exhale and twist up through your upper spine.

9 Turn your head to look over your right shoulder.

10 Hold the pose for 30 seconds to 1 minute and then return to Seated Mountain Pose.

11 Repeat steps 1 to 10 for your other side.

Chapter 7

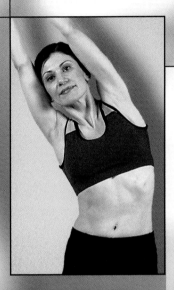

Standing poses are beneficial for improving your posture, strengthening your legs and stretching your entire body. Some standing poses serve as starting positions for other poses, so it is important to learn these core poses. This chapter takes you through several standing poses you can perform as part of your yoga practice. It is important to concentrate on your alignment in these standing poses to achieve the full benefits of the poses.

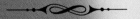

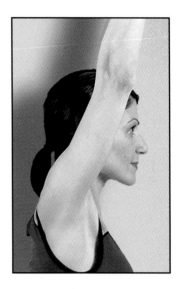

Standing Poses

In this Chapter...

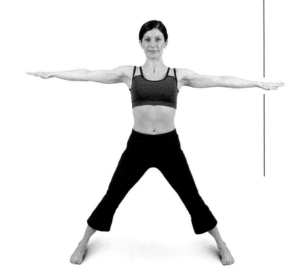

mountain pose *(tadasana)*

Mountain Pose is a basic standing pose that can help you improve your posture, stability and balance. This pose serves as a starting position for all other standing poses.

Practicing Mountain Pose will teach you how to correctly align your body when standing. When your body is aligned correctly, your head, neck and spine form a straight line.

While in Mountain Pose, picture your body divided into two halves—one half below your waist and the other half above your waist. Your lower body should feel stable and grounded and your upper body should feel light and relaxed. To achieve this feeling, you can visualize your head and torso rising away from your legs and feet.

Since Mountain Pose seems simple, you may be tempted to rush through the pose. Instead, you should take time to relax, remain still and breathe evenly. Taking your time will allow you to achieve the full benefits of the pose.

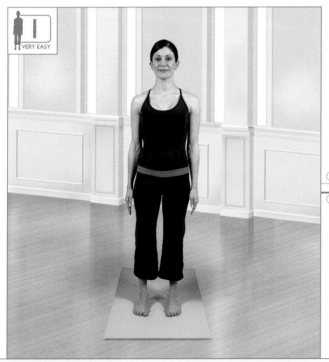

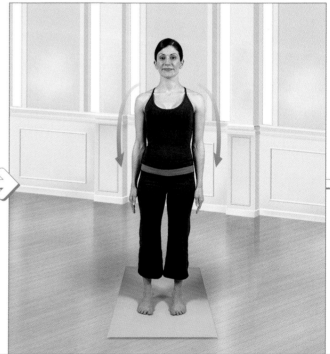

1 Stand tall and relaxed with your feet hip width apart.

2 Inhale as you lift and spread your toes and then place them softly on the floor.

3 Balance your weight between the soles of your feet and allow your toes to relax.

- Your legs and feet should feel grounded and stable.

4 Tuck your tailbone under to lengthen your spine.

5 Relax your shoulders down and allow your arms to hang by your sides with your palms facing your legs.

- Your upper body should feel light and relaxed.

How can I determine if my weight is properly balanced in this pose?

Finding the proper balance of your weight is an important part of Mountain Pose. To determine if your weight is properly balanced, rock back and forth and side to side on your feet, noticing the difference in the distribution of your weight. When your weight feels evenly distributed between the soles of both of your feet, stop rocking and remain still. Remember to keep your toes relaxed as your weight rests on the soles of your feet.

How can I determine if my body is aligned correctly?

While performing Mountain Pose, stand with the back of your head, your buttocks and your heels touching a wall or the edge of a doorway. This can help you determine if your body is aligned correctly. As you continue to practice Mountain Pose, your head will automatically come to balance at the top of your spine when your body is aligned correctly.

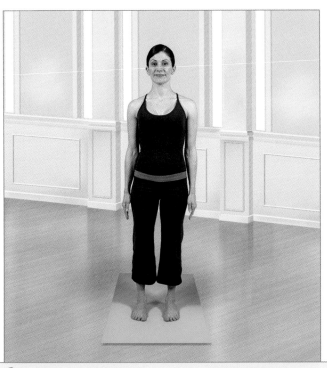

MODIFICATION

6 Point the crown of your head toward the ceiling and gaze at a fixed point in front of you.

7 Relax your face, eyes, jaw and throat.

• Visualize your head and torso rising away from your legs and feet.

8 Hold the pose for 30 seconds to 1 minute.

• You can perform Mountain Pose with your arms extended over your head. This modification stretches your arms and shoulders.

1 After holding Mountain Pose, inhale as you raise your arms above your head, keeping your shoulders relaxed down. Your arms should be shoulder width apart and your palms should be facing each other. Hold the pose for another 30 seconds to 1 minute.

five pointed star pose

You can perform Five Pointed Star Pose to energize and lengthen your entire body. This pose also opens your chest, which can help improve your circulation and capacity for deep breathing. Performing Five Pointed Star Pose can also help to correctly align your spine. You may want to use this pose as a starting position for Triangle Pose or Standing Wide Angle Forward Bend.

As you hold Five Pointed Star Pose, visualize your body stretching and lengthening in all five directions at

once—through the crown of your head and through each arm and leg. You should also focus on breathing evenly. As you inhale, feel your breath coming into the center of your body. As you exhale, feel your breath radiating out through the crown of your head, your fingertips and the soles of your feet.

If your arms or shoulders feel strained in this pose, you can place your hands on your hips.

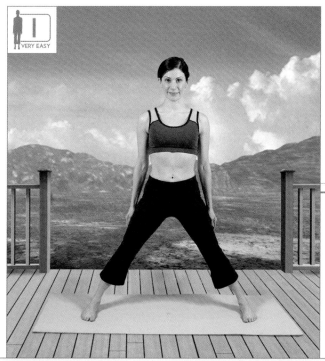

VERY EASY

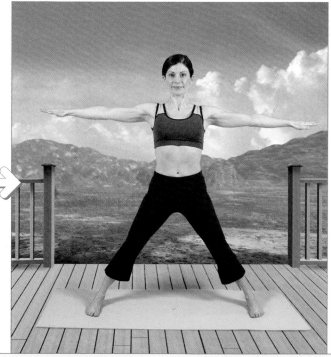

1 Begin in Mountain Pose. For information on Mountain Pose, see page 120.

2 Step your right foot to the right 3 to 5 feet.

- Make sure your feet are parallel and your toes are pointing straight ahead.

3 Raise your arms to shoulder height at your sides, with your palms facing down.

4 Relax your shoulders down and back.

5 Tuck your tailbone under to help prevent your lower back from over-arching.

6 Press your feet into the floor and press the crown of your head toward the ceiling. Extend through your fingertips.

7 Hold the pose for 30 seconds to 1 minute and then return to Mountain Pose.

goddess pose

Goddess Pose, also known as Victory Squat, opens your chest and hips, while strengthening your lower body. You can use this pose to warm up and energize your entire body.

Practicing Goddess Pose can help you feel empowered, as well as build your self-discipline. Try to focus on honoring your feminine energy as you hold the pose. As you breathe in Goddess Pose, visualize the spirit of a goddess coursing through your body.

Once you feel comfortable performing Goddess Pose, you can deepen the pose by moving your sitting bones closer to the floor. When deepening the pose, make sure you do not overextend your knees.

If you find Goddess Pose places too much strain on your arms and shoulders, you can rest your palms on your thighs. Make sure you use caution performing this pose if you have a leg, hip, back or shoulder injury.

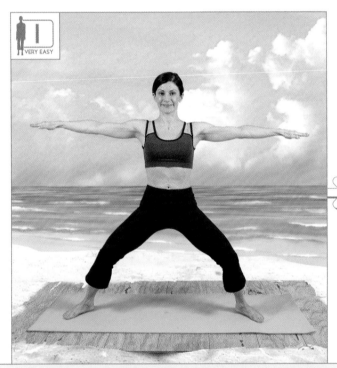
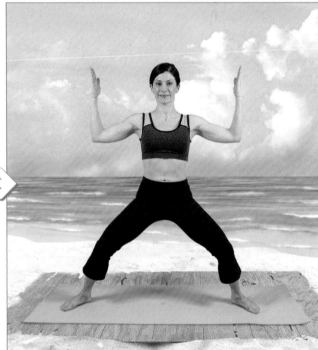

VERY EASY

1 Begin in Five Pointed Star Pose. For information on Five Pointed Star Pose, see page 122.

2 Turn your right foot to the right 45 degrees and turn your left foot to the left 45 degrees.

3 Bend your knees and lower your hips toward the floor. Your knees should not extend past your toes.

4 Tilt your pelvis under to lengthen your spine.

5 Bend your elbows and point your fingertips toward the ceiling.

6 Turn your palms to face your body.

• Your elbows should be pointing toward the floor and should be slightly lower than your shoulders.

7 Point the crown of your head toward the ceiling and gaze straight ahead.

8 Hold the pose for 30 seconds to 1 minute and then return to Five Pointed Star Pose.

crescent moon pose *(ardha chandrasana)*

Crescent Moon Pose is an energizing pose that opens and stretches the sides of your body. Regular practice of this pose builds core body strength, increases the flexibility of your spine and improves circulation.

As you move into this pose, you should focus on lengthening your body, rather than stretching as far to the side as you can. You may find it helpful to visualize the lengthening of the side of your body from your ankle to your fingertips. To warm up your body before

holding Crescent Moon Pose, you can perform the pose by moving from side to side twice.

While holding the pose, keep your shoulders relaxed down and back so that your face, chest and hips are open to the front. You should also make sure that you do not compress the side of your body that your arms are leaning over.

Use caution performing Crescent Moon Pose if you have lower back or shoulder problems.

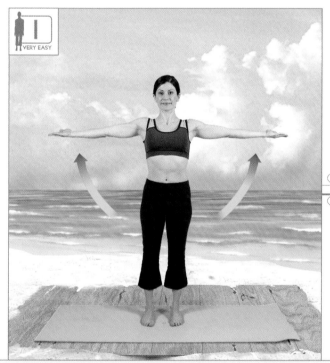

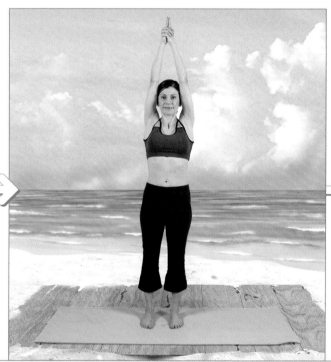

VERY EASY

1 Begin in Mountain Pose. For information on Mountain Pose, see page 120.

2 Raise your arms to shoulder height at your sides.

3 Turn your palms to face the ceiling.

4 Inhale and bring your hands together over your head.

5 Interlace your fingers and point your index fingers toward the ceiling.

• Your shoulders should be relaxed down and back.

• Make sure you keep your upper arms beside your ears throughout the pose.

How can I reduce the stress on my lower back in this pose?

To reduce the stress on your lower back, begin the pose with your feet slightly further than hip width apart. Also, do not press your hips to the side as described in step **8** below. This modification is also useful for keeping your hips stable in the pose.

I find this pose strains my shoulders. What can I do?

Place your right hand on your right hip and raise your left arm up over your head. Then lean to the right to stretch your left side. Repeat for your other side.

How can I make sure my chest and pelvis are open in this pose?

To ensure your chest and pelvis are open, practice this pose with your shoulder blades and buttocks lightly touching a wall.

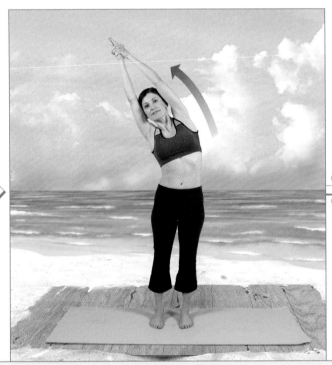

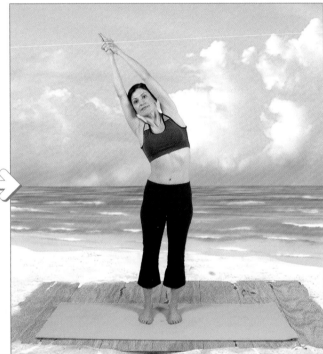

6 Inhale and press the soles of your feet into the floor as you extend up through your fingertips.

7 Exhale and bend from the waist as you lean to the right.

8 Press your hips gently to the left.

- Make sure you are pressing evenly through both feet.

9 Point the crown of your head toward your hands and gaze straight ahead.

10 Hold the pose for 15 to 30 seconds.

11 Inhale as you return your torso to an upright position.

12 Repeat steps 6 to 11 for your other side.

- To come out of the pose, exhale as you bring your arms to your sides.

chair pose *(utkatasana)*

Chair Pose is a standing pose that strengthens your lower body and torso. This pose also stretches your shoulders and opens your chest.

As you bend your knees to lower your hips in this pose, allow your torso to lean over your thighs slightly. However, your torso should remain as upright as possible, keeping your head aligned with your spine. You can deepen Chair Pose by lowering your hips a bit further, but you should not feel any strain in your knees or lower back. Make sure you do not lower your

hips below your knees or allow your knees to extend past your toes. You should be able to look down and see your toes.

While performing the pose, make sure you keep your feet firmly planted on the floor. Your legs should feel stable and grounded. You should also concentrate on breathing deeply and evenly to help release any tension in your legs or any other part of your body.

Use caution performing Chair Pose if you have hip or knee problems.

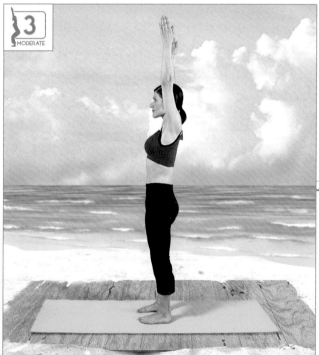

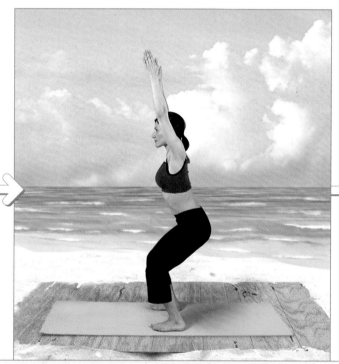

1 Begin in Mountain Pose. For information on Mountain Pose, see page 120.

2 Inhale as you raise your arms above your head, with your palms facing each other, shoulder width apart.

• Make sure your shoulders and arms are relaxed. Your arms should be straight, but your elbows should not be locked.

3 Exhale as you bend your knees as if you were about to sit in a chair until you feel a comfortable stretch in the front of your thighs. Do not lower your hips below your knees.

• Make sure your heels stay on the floor.

4 Tuck your tailbone under to protect your lower back from arching.

My lower back feels strained in Chair Pose. What can I do?

You can place your hands on the top of your thighs as you perform the pose. This modification can ease the strain in your lower back by supporting the weight of your body with your arms.

How can I stretch my arms and upper body more in Chair Pose?

Perform the pose as described below, except interlace your fingers above your head and then rotate your wrists so your palms face the ceiling. Then stretch your arms toward the ceiling.

I find it difficult to hold Chair Pose. How can I modify the pose to give me more stability?

If you have difficulty holding Chair Pose, you can perform the pose using a wall for support. Stand approximately one foot away from a wall with your back to the wall. As you bend your knees to move into the pose, your tailbone should lightly touch the wall. You may need to adjust your distance from the wall to ensure you are in the correct position.

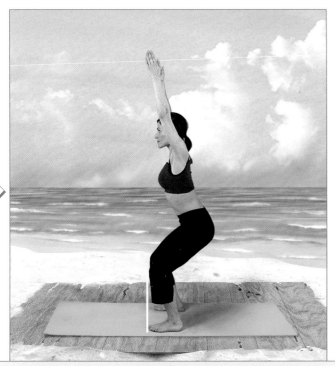

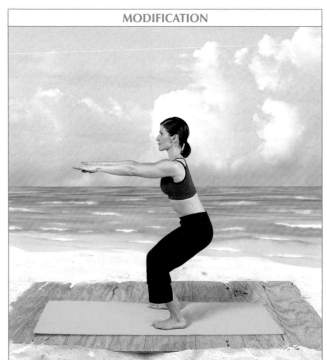

MODIFICATION

• Make sure your knees do not extend past your toes and your knees are hip width apart.

5 Point the crown of your head toward the ceiling and gaze straight ahead.

6 Hold the pose for 10 seconds to 1 minute.

7 To come out of the pose, inhale as you straighten your legs. Then exhale as you bring your arms back down to your sides. Return to Mountain Pose.

• You can perform Chair Pose with your arms extended in front of you. This modification is easier on your shoulders and arms and can also help you maintain your balance.

1 Perform Chair Pose, except raise your arms to shoulder height in front of you, instead of above your head.

warrior I pose *(virabhadrasana I)*

Warrior I Pose is a standing pose that strengthens your legs and stretches your arms and shoulders, while opening your chest. This pose can also help increase your stamina and improve your balance. Named after the mythic warrior *Virabhadra*, Warrior I Pose promotes a feeling of strength and power.

While performing this pose, make sure your head, shoulders, hips and knees all face the same direction. As you hold the pose, visualize the smooth line of your body from the heel of your back foot to your fingertips.

To help you feel grounded and stable in this pose, make sure both of your feet are in even contact with the floor, supporting the weight of your body. If you still find it difficult to balance, you can turn your back foot out on a slight angle. If your lower back feels strained in this pose, you can lean your torso forward slightly over your bent leg.

You should use caution performing Warrior I Pose if you have hip, knee, back or shoulder problems.

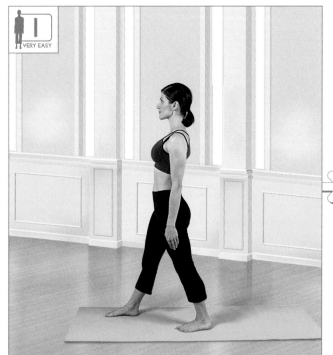
VERY EASY

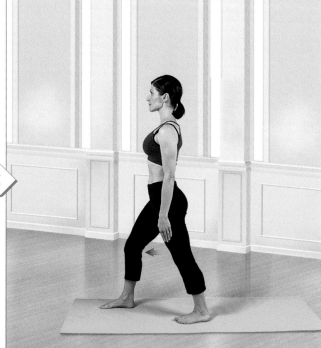

1 Begin in Mountain Pose. For information on Mountain Pose, see page 120.

2 Step your right foot forward 2 to 4 feet. Your feet should be hip width apart, with your toes pointing forward.

3 Bend your right knee slightly.

- Your left leg should be straight and the sole of your left foot should be firmly planted on the floor.

- Make sure your weight is evenly distributed between both feet.

4 Face your head, shoulders, hips and knees forward.

How can I vary the position of my arms in this pose?

There are several positions you can choose for your arms in this pose. You can raise your arms above your head and grasp your elbows with the opposite hands. You can also extend your arms out to the sides, with your palms facing down. If you have shoulder problems, you can place your hands on your hips.

Is there a more advanced variation of Warrior I Pose?

Yes. While holding the pose, bring your palms together, keeping your arms stretched up toward the ceiling. Then tilt your head back to look up at the ceiling. As you become more flexible, you can perform a back bend in this pose. To perform a back bend, move your hands back slightly, as you gently arch your back and tilt your head to look up and back. Remember to maintain length through your spine and neck. You should not allow your head to drop back.

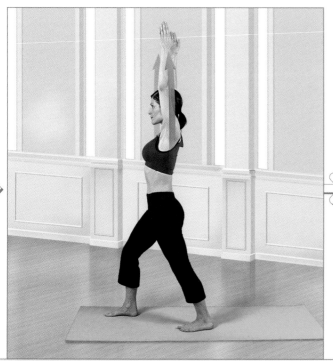

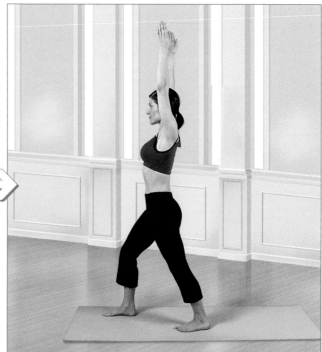

5 Inhale as you raise your arms above your head, palms facing each other and fingers pointing toward the ceiling.

6 Relax your shoulders down away from your ears.

7 Point the crown of your head toward the ceiling and gaze straight ahead.

8 Hold the pose for 15 seconds to 1 minute.

9 To come out of the pose, exhale as you lower your arms to your sides. Then return to Mountain Pose.

10 Repeat steps 2 to 9 for your other side.

warrior II pose *(virabhadrasana II)*

Warrior II Pose strengthens and stretches your legs, ankles, shoulders and arms. This pose also expands your chest, which can help you breathe more deeply. Regular practice of this pose can increase your strength and stamina.

To avoid arching your lower back in the pose, tuck your tailbone under. You should also make sure that the hip of your back leg does not rotate forward. Your arms, shoulders, hips and legs should all be on the same plane. You should also keep your bent knee directly over your ankle to avoid overextending your knee.

As you hold the pose, your lower body should feel grounded through both feet. Try to visualize your legs as pillars of strength that support your expanding chest and stretching arms.

If you have neck problems, do not turn your head to gaze out over your hand. Instead, keep your neck straight and look forward. You should also use caution performing this pose if you have hip or knee problems.

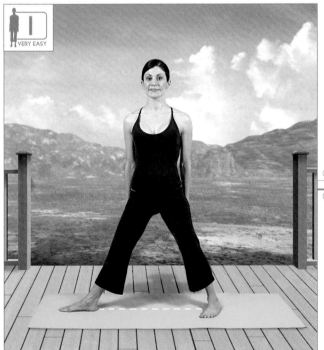

VERY EASY

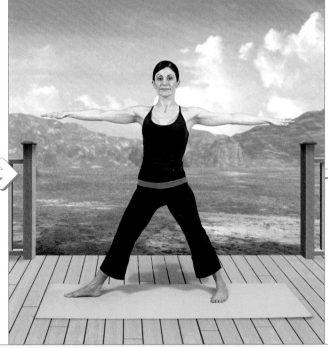

1 Begin in Mountain Pose. For information on Mountain Pose, see page 120.

2 Step your right foot to the right 2 to 4 feet.

3 Turn your right foot out 90 degrees and then turn your left foot in 45 degrees.

- Make sure your right heel is aligned with the middle of your left foot.

- Your shoulders and hips should be facing forward on the same plane as your legs.

4 Tuck your tailbone under to avoid arching your lower back.

5 Inhale as you raise your arms up to shoulder height, with your palms facing down.

6 Relax your shoulders down and back away from your ears.

How can I intensify the stretch in my arms in Warrior II Pose?

You can rotate your arms and hands until your palms and the inside of your elbows face the ceiling. While maintaining the rotation of your arms, use your wrists to turn your palms toward the floor again.

How can I modify the pose if my arms become tired?

If your arms become tired, you can place your hands on your hips instead of raising your arms up to shoulder height.

I find it difficult to balance in Warrior II Pose. What can I do?

You can use a wall to help you balance in this pose. Begin the pose standing with your back facing a wall with both heels against the wall. Step your right foot forward 2 to 4 feet and turn your left foot out so the left side of your foot is against the wall to provide stability for the pose. Then perform the pose as described below, except place your hands on your hips instead of raising your arms to shoulder height.

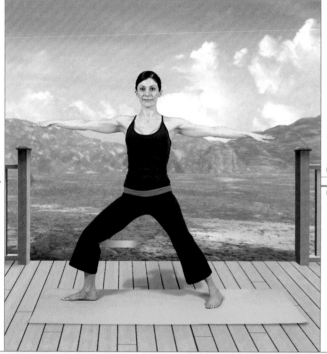

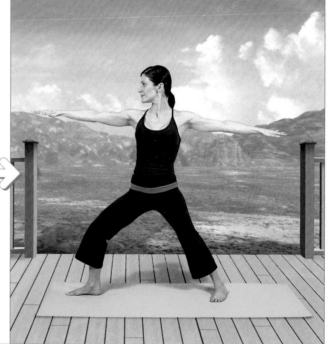

7 Exhale as you bend your right knee until it is over your right ankle. Your right knee should be facing the same direction as your toes.

• Make sure your left leg is straight and the soles of both feet are in even contact with the floor.

8 Turn your head to the right and gaze out over the fingertips of your right hand.

9 Hold the pose for 30 seconds to 1 minute.

10 To come out of the pose, exhale as you lower your arms to your sides and straighten your right leg. Then return to Mountain Pose.

11 Repeat steps 2 to 10 for your other side.

side angle pose *(parsvakonasana)*

Side Angle Pose provides an intense stretch along the sides of your body, with an emphasis on stretching the sides of your waist and rib cage. You can practice this pose to strengthen and increase the flexibility of your hips, legs and ankles. This pose also opens your chest, which can help increase your lung capacity.

As you perform Side Angle Pose, keep your front knee over your ankle and the outer edge of your back foot in contact with the floor. Even though your weight

will fall mostly on your front foot in this pose, try to center your weight as much as possible.

Proper body alignment is important in this pose. Keep your spine straight and your head, shoulders and hips on the same plane. To help align your body correctly, you can perform the pose with your back against a wall.

You should be very careful performing Side Angle Pose if you have lower back problems. If you have a stiff neck, do not look up at the ceiling in the pose.

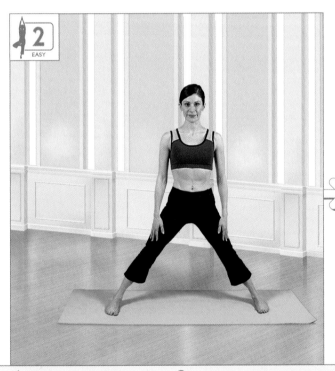

1 Begin in Mountain Pose. For information on Mountain Pose, see page 120.

2 Step your right foot to the right approximately 3 feet.

3 Turn your left foot in 45 degrees and then turn your right foot out 90 degrees.

- Make sure your right heel is aligned with the middle of your left foot.

4 Inhale as you raise your arms up to shoulder height, with your palms facing down. Your arms and shoulders should be relaxed.

I cannot place my palm on the floor in Side Angle Pose. What can I do?

Unless you are very flexible, it may be difficult for you to place your palm on the floor in this pose. Try placing your palm on the inside of your front foot instead of the outside. You can also touch the floor with your fingertips instead of your palm. If you still cannot reach the floor, position a block on the outside of your front foot and then rest your palm on the block.

I feel strain in my legs and lower back while performing this pose. How can I modify the pose to reduce the strain?

To reduce the strain in your legs and lower back, you can place your elbow on your front thigh, with your forearm parallel to the floor, instead of placing your palm on the floor. Resting your elbow on your thigh can also help you maintain proper body alignment.

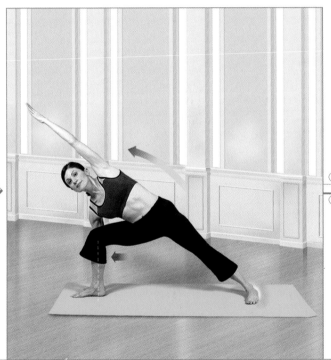

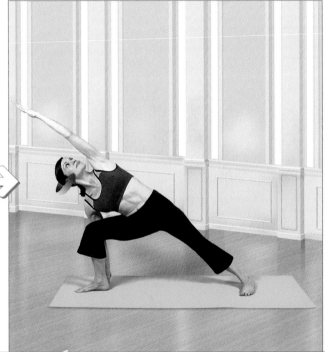

5 Bend your right knee until it is over your right ankle.

6 Exhale as you bend your torso to the right and place the palm of your right hand on the floor outside your right foot.

• Make sure your left leg is straight and the outer edge of your left foot is in contact with the floor.

7 Stretch your left arm over your head, keeping your left shoulder back.

8 Turn your head and look at the ceiling, keeping your spine straight and your neck relaxed.

9 Hold the pose for 10 to 20 seconds.

10 To come out of the pose, press your right foot into the floor and then inhale as you lift your right palm off the floor and straighten your right leg. Then return to Mountain Pose.

11 Repeat steps 2 to 10 for your other side.

triangle pose *(trikonasana)*

Triangle Pose provides an intense stretch along the sides of your torso, hips and legs. With regular practice of this pose, you can increase the strength and flexibility of your hips, legs, ankles and feet. This pose also elongates your spine and opens your chest, which can help improve your breathing.

It is important to be aware of the alignment of your body in Triangle Pose. Make sure your head, shoulders and hips are on the same plane. You must also keep your spine in a straight line from your head down to

your tailbone. Practicing the pose with your back against a wall can help you find the proper alignment.

As you rest your weight on your back heel in this pose, you should feel stable and grounded through both of your feet. You should also feel comfortable in the pose, with your neck relaxed, your knees soft and your legs stretched, but not strained.

Use caution performing Triangle Pose if you have lower back problems.

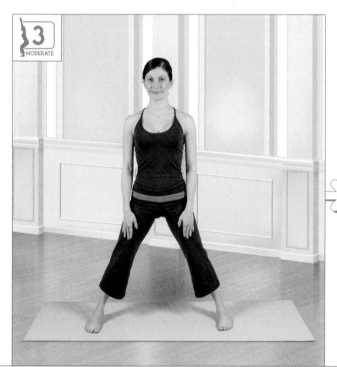

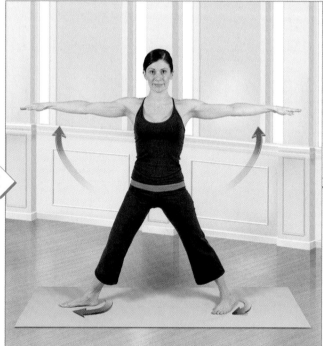

1 Begin in Mountain Pose. For information on Mountain Pose, see page 120.

2 Step your right foot to the right 3 to 5 feet.

3 Turn your left foot in 45 degrees and then turn your right foot out 90 degrees.

- Make sure your right heel is aligned with the middle of your left foot.

4 Inhale as you raise your arms up to shoulder height, with your palms facing down. Your arms and shoulders should be relaxed.

What should I do if my palm cannot reach the floor?

If your palm cannot reach the floor in this pose, you can place your palm on the ankle, shin or knee of your front leg. You can also position a block on the outside of your front foot and place your palm on the block. Trying to force your palm to the floor may cause your body to become improperly aligned. Achieving correct body alignment is more important than trying to reach down as far as possible.

I have a stiff neck and cannot look up in Triangle Pose. Can I still perform the pose?

You can still perform Triangle Pose, but you should look down at the floor instead of looking up at your raised hand. With a stiff neck, you may also have problems finding a comfortable position for your raised arm. To reduce the strain on your neck, rest the hand of your raised arm on your hip instead of stretching it toward the ceiling.

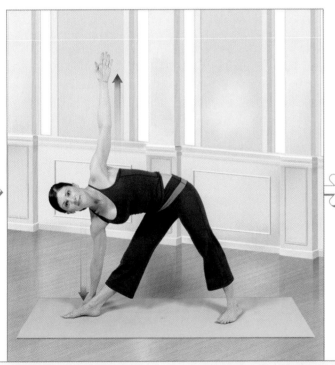

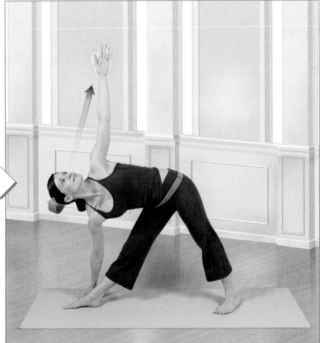

5 Shift your hips to the left and extend your upper body to the right.

6 Exhale as you place the palm of your right hand on the floor outside your right foot.

• If you cannot reach the floor, you can place your palm on your lower leg.

7 Stretch your left arm up toward the ceiling, with your palm facing forward.

• Make sure you keep your left shoulder back.

8 Turn your head to look up at your left hand, keeping your spine straight and your neck relaxed.

9 Hold the pose for 10 to 30 seconds.

10 To come out of the pose, press the soles of your feet into the floor and then inhale as you lift your right palm off the floor. Then return to Mountain Pose.

11 Repeat steps 2 to 10 for your other side.

Chapter 8

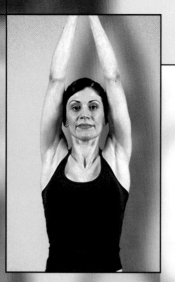

Standing balancing poses are great for improving your balance, coordination and concentration. Performing standing balancing poses can also help you develop the ability to remain grounded in all types of poses. Although some standing balancing poses are challenging, they are very rewarding. You should try to incorporate the standing balancing poses in this chapter into your yoga practice.

Standing Balancing Poses

In this Chapter...

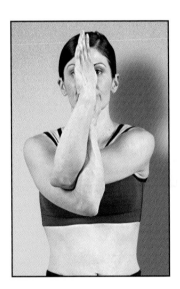

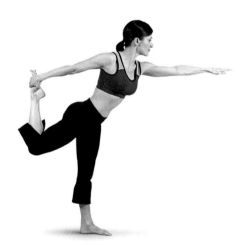

stork
pose

You can perform Stork Pose to improve your balance and stability. This pose also helps to open your hips and strengthen your legs, arms and shoulders. If you are feeling distracted or unfocused, you can perform Stork Pose to center and focus your mind.

You may find it easier to balance on one side of your body than the other side. You may also find that on some days it is easier to balance in this pose than on other days. Balancing poses reflect the balancing of your body, mind and spirit, so difficulty balancing in

this pose on a particular day may be a reflection of an imbalance elsewhere in your life.

Try coming in and out of the pose a few times to develop your balance. Once you find your balance, you can remain steady in the pose by sinking your weight down through your supporting foot, gazing at a fixed point in front of you and breathing evenly.

As you hold Stork Pose, resist the temptation to lean forward. Instead, focus on keeping your spine straight and lengthened.

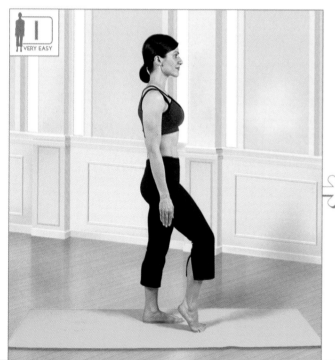

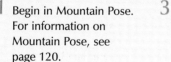

VERY EASY

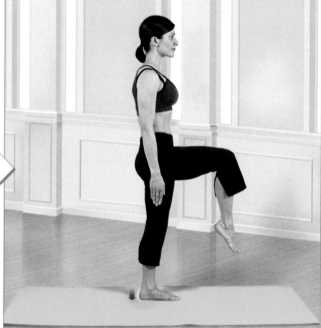

1 Begin in Mountain Pose. For information on Mountain Pose, see page 120.

2 Shift your weight onto your left leg and foot.

3 Bend your right leg and lift your right heel off the floor.

4 Bring your right knee up until your thigh is parallel to the floor. Your leg should form a 90-degree angle.

• Make sure your lower right leg is perpendicular to the floor and your toes are pointing toward the floor.

5 Press the heel of your left foot into the floor.

What can I do if I have difficulty maintaining my balance?

You can stand beside a wall and place one hand on the wall for support while performing the pose. Once you feel stable, you can remove your hand from the wall.

How can I make Stork Pose more challenging?

Stretch your arms above your head so your upper arms are beside your ears and your palms are facing each other. Make sure you keep your shoulders relaxed and down.

What should I do if the hip of my raised leg moves when I bend my knee?

Instead of raising your arms in front of you, you should rest your hands on your hips so that you can feel any movement in your hips. If you feel your hip rise, reduce the bend in your knee slightly. Resting your hands on your hips in this pose can also help improve your balance.

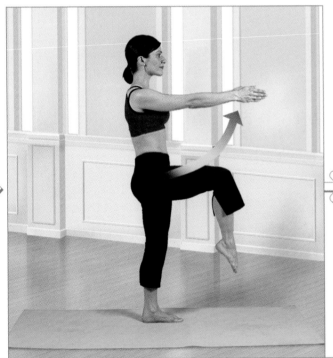

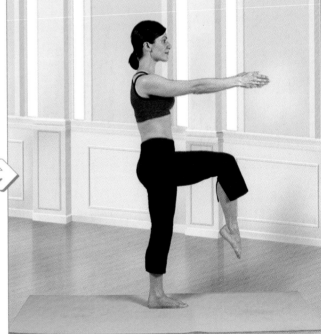

6 Inhale as you raise your arms to shoulder height in front of you.

• Your arms should be straight, but your elbows should not be locked.

7 Turn your palms to face each other and stretch out through your fingertips.

8 Relax your shoulders down away from your ears.

9 Point the crown of your head toward the ceiling and gaze at a fixed point in front of you.

10 Hold the pose for 15 seconds to 1 minute and then return to Mountain Pose.

11 Repeat steps 2 to 10 for your other side.

dancer pose *(natarajasana)*

Dancer Pose, also known as Lord of the Dance Pose, can help improve your balance and stability. This pose also helps to open your chest and strengthen your shoulders, arms and legs.

You may want to perform Dancer Pose to stretch your shoulders, back, hips and legs after you have spent all day sitting in a chair. If you are feeling distracted or unfocused, you can perform Dancer Pose to help improve your ability to concentrate.

Once you feel comfortable and balanced in the pose, you can try deepening the pose slightly by leaning forward more and stretching your raised leg up higher. Deepening the pose in this way will intensify the stretch and further challenge your balance. As you perform this pose, visualize yourself as a dancer radiating poise and grace.

You should be careful performing Dancer Pose if you have problems with your back, shoulders, hips or knees.

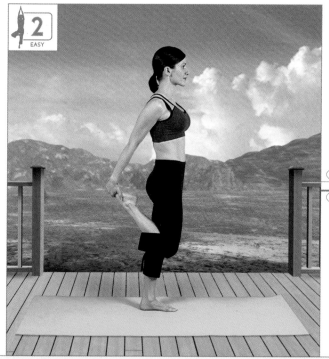

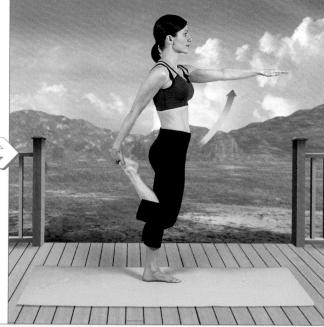

1 Begin in Mountain Pose. For information on Mountain Pose, see page 120.

2 Shift your weight onto your left leg and foot and bend your right knee slightly to lift your right heel off the floor.

3 Bend your right knee and bring your right leg behind you.

4 Reach behind you with your right hand and clasp your right ankle or the top of your right foot.

- Make sure your knees are together and parallel with each other.

5 Raise your left arm to shoulder height in front of you, with your palm facing down.

- Make sure your shoulders are relaxed and your arms are straight, but your elbows are not locked.

I have difficulty balancing in Dancer Pose. What can I do?

If you find it difficult to balance in this pose, only perform steps 1 to 5 below before holding the pose. Then repeat these steps for your other side. If you are still having trouble balancing, you can perform this variation using a wall for support. Stand beside a wall and raise your arm out to the side to place your hand on the wall for support.

What can I do if I cannot reach my foot in this pose?

Loop a strap around the top of your foot and then grasp the ends of the strap in your hand. Keep the strap taut, but do not use the strap to pull yourself into the pose.

How can I intensify the stretch in Dancer Pose?

To perform a more advanced version of Dancer Pose, you can reach your arm over your head to hold your foot behind you.

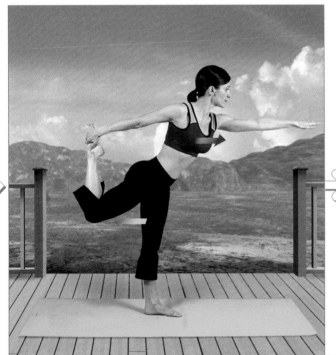

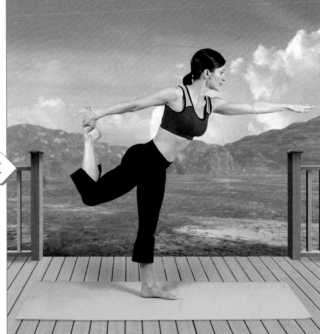

6 Exhale as you press your left foot into the floor and lean your torso slightly forward.

7 Stretch your right leg away from your body and press your foot into your hand.

• Keep your right knee directly behind you. Do not allow your knee to turn to the side.

• Make sure your chest and hips are facing forward.

8 Allow your head and neck to follow the curve of your spine.

9 Hold the pose for 15 to 30 seconds.

10 To come out of the pose, bring your torso back to an upright position. Then release your right leg and return to Mountain Pose.

11 Repeat steps 2 to 10 for your other side.

tree
pose *(vrksasana)*

Tree Pose is a standing balancing pose that provides a good stretch to your entire body. The pose can also strengthen your legs, ankles and feet and help increase the flexibility of your hips and knees.

To perform Tree Pose, you bend one leg and place the sole of your foot against the inside of your other leg. Standing on one foot, you then stretch your arms above your head. While in the pose, try to visualize your body stretching downward through your

supporting leg, upward through your arms and outward through your bent leg.

You may find it difficult to maintain your balance in this pose. To remain steady, sink your weight down through your supporting foot. Imagine your supporting foot as a root that keeps you solidly planted in the ground. Gazing at a fixed point in front of you and breathing evenly can also help you maintain your balance. Make sure you take your time performing Tree Pose. It may take you a while to find your balance.

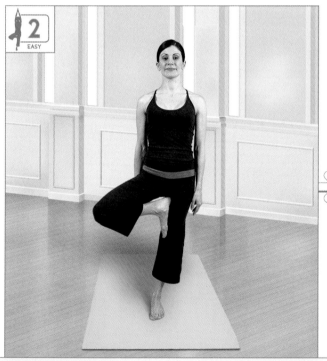

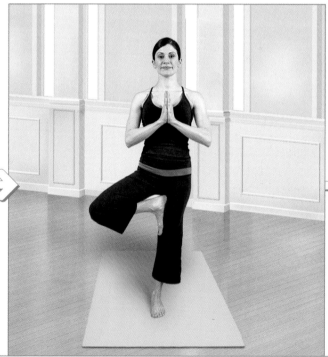

1 Begin in Mountain Pose. For information on Mountain Pose, see page 120.

2 Shift your weight onto your left foot and then bend your right leg.

3 Place the sole of your right foot against the inside of your left leg as high up as is comfortable. Do not place your foot against your knee joint.

- Point the toes on your right foot toward the floor.

4 Bring your palms together at chest level in Prayer Pose.

5 Press the sole of your right foot firmly against the inside of your left leg and relax your bent right leg away from your hip.

What can I do if I have difficulty maintaining my balance?

If you find you cannot maintain your balance in Tree Pose, you can stand beside a wall and place one hand on the wall for support while performing the pose. Once you feel stable, you can remove your hand from the wall and raise your arm above your head. You can also steady yourself by standing with your shoulder blades and buttocks against a wall as you perform the pose. When you are confident in your ability to remain balanced in Tree Pose, try performing the pose away from a wall.

How can I make Tree Pose more challenging?

You can perform Tree Pose with your eyes closed to make the pose more challenging. When you do not gaze at a fixed point in front of you, you challenge your ability to remain balanced. In addition to keeping your body balanced, closing your eyes can challenge you to focus your mind.

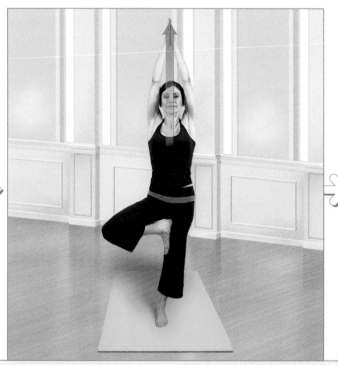

6 Press the sole of your left foot into the floor.

7 Inhale as you raise your arms above your head, keeping your palms together, and stretch out through your fingertips.

8 Point the crown of your head toward the ceiling and gaze at a fixed point in front of you.

• Visualize yourself stretching in three different directions at once—downward, upward and outward.

9 Hold the pose for 15 to 30 seconds and then return to Mountain Pose.

10 Repeat steps 2 to 9 for your other side.

standing hand
to toe pose *(utthita hasta padangusthasana)*

Standing Hand to Toe Pose provides a good stretch to your hips, hamstrings, calves and ankles. This is a challenging pose that requires you to use strength, flexibility and coordination to remain balanced on your supporting leg. As you work on keeping your body balanced in Standing Hand to Toe Pose, you may improve your concentration and mental focus.

As you hold the pose, try to resist the temptation to lean forward. Instead, focus on keeping your spine straight and lengthened. If you find that you cannot fully straighten your leg in this pose, try to straighten your leg as much as you can without compromising your balance or the upright position of your torso. To improve your balance in Standing Hand to Toe Pose, sink your weight down through your supporting foot and gaze at a fixed point in front of you.

You should use caution performing this pose if you have an arm, leg or shoulder injury.

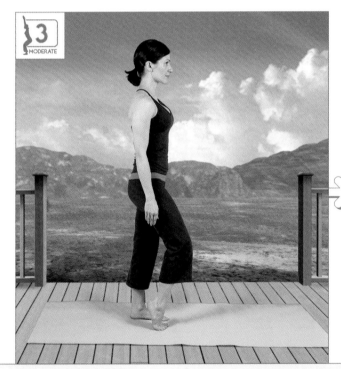

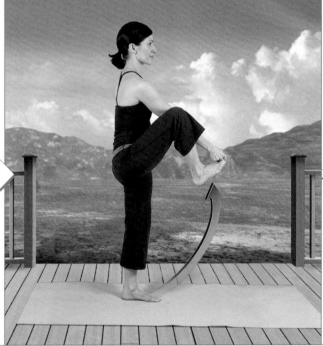

1 Begin in Mountain Pose. For information on Mountain Pose, see page 120.

2 Rest your left hand on your left hip.

3 Bend your right leg and lift your right heel off the floor.

4 Shift your weight onto your left leg and foot.

5 Bring your right knee up in front of you.

6 Wrap the middle finger, index finger and thumb of your right hand around the big toe of your right foot.

7 Press the heel of your left foot into the floor.

What can I do if I find it difficult to straighten my leg in this pose?

You can loop a yoga strap around the foot of your extended leg to perform the pose. If you do not have a yoga strap, you can use any cloth strap, such as a bathrobe belt. Make sure you do not pull on the strap. You should use the strap only to support your leg.

How can I deepen the pose?

To deepen the pose, bring your extended leg out to your side. For example, if your right leg is extended, bring your right leg out to your right side. When your arm and leg are extended to your side, your arm should be parallel to the floor. Make sure you keep your hips level while performing this modification.

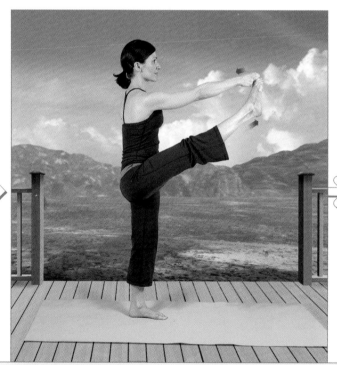

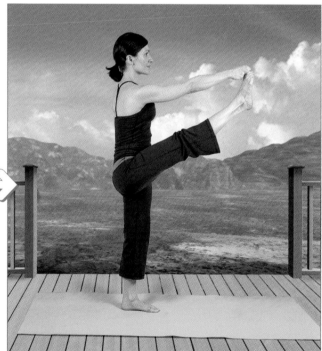

8 Inhale as you slowly straighten your right leg in front of you.

9 Press out through your right heel as you gently pull your toe toward your body.

- Make sure your shoulders are relaxed back and down.

10 Point the crown of your head toward the ceiling and gaze at a fixed point in front of you.

11 Hold the pose for 15 seconds to 1 minute and then return to Mountain Pose.

12 Repeat steps 2 to 11 for your other side.

eagle pose *(garudasana)*

Eagle Pose helps to improve your balance and provides a good stretch to your upper back, shoulders and outer thighs. With regular practice of this pose, you can also strengthen your legs, knees and ankles.

To perform Eagle Pose, you wrap one leg around the other, which helps to open the back of your pelvis, and one arm around the other, which helps to create space between your shoulder blades.

As you perform Eagle Pose, you should focus on keeping your spine straight and your hips and shoulders facing forward.

When you first start practicing this pose, you may find it difficult to maintain your balance. Breathing evenly and gazing at a fixed point 4 or 5 feet in front of you can help you maintain your balance. Do not be tempted to grip the floor or mat with your toes. This will only make balancing more difficult.

You should be careful performing Eagle Pose if you have shoulder, arm, hip or knee problems.

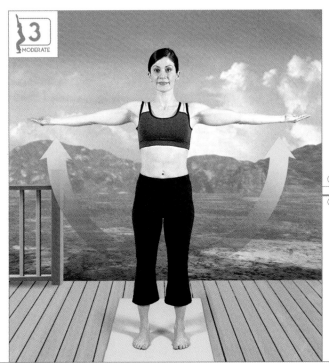

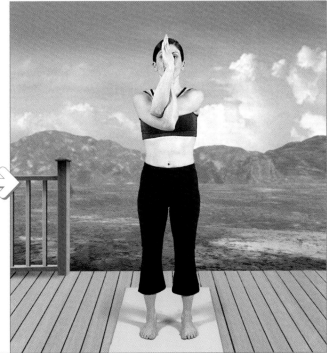

1 Begin in Mountain Pose. For information on Mountain Pose, see page 120.

2 Inhale as you raise your arms up to shoulder height at your sides, with your palms facing up. Your arms and shoulders should be relaxed.

3 Cross your left arm over your right arm so your elbows are on top of each other.

4 Bend your elbows and wrap your forearms around each other so your palms are facing each other.

• Make sure your fingers are pointing toward the ceiling.

• If your palms do not touch, rest one palm against your other wrist or forearm.

I cannot wrap my arms around one another. How should I position my arms?

If have shoulder or arm problems, you can position your arms in Prayer Pose. For information on Prayer Pose, see page 48.

How can I increase the stretch in my shoulders and arms?

After you wrap your arms around one another, you can lift your hands and arms up toward the ceiling to increase the stretch. Lift your hands up only as far as is comfortable for you and keep your shoulders down. You should not feel any strain in your shoulders.

I have problems balancing in Eagle Pose. What can I do?

You can try performing the pose with your back lightly touching a wall. If you still find the balancing aspect of this pose too difficult, you can stand in Mountain Pose and perform only the arm movements in steps 3 and 4 below. This will allow you to remain balanced and still perform a great shoulder stretch.

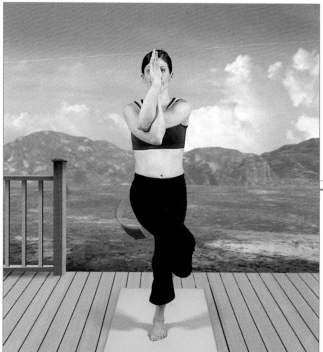

5 Bend your knees slightly and then shift your weight to your left leg.

6 Cross your right leg over your left leg just above your left knee.

7 Move your right foot behind your left lower leg and hook your foot over your left calf muscle or ankle.

• If you cannot reach your left calf muscle, position your right foot beside your left lower leg.

8 Point the crown of your head toward the ceiling and gaze straight ahead.

• Visualize the straight line of your spine running the length of your body.

9 Hold the pose for 30 seconds to 1 minute and then return to Mountain Pose.

10 Repeat steps 2 to 9, crossing your opposite arm and leg over in steps 3 and 6.

half moon pose *(ardha chandrasana)*

Half Moon Pose is an advanced standing balancing pose that stretches your body in several directions at once—out through your legs, the crown of your head and your arms. This pose can strengthen your legs and buttocks, as well as increase the flexibility of your legs and hips. Regular practice of Half Moon Pose can also improve your balance and coordination.

To help maintain your balance in this pose, rest your weight on your supporting foot as you press it into the floor and extend your raised leg away from you with each exhalation. Concentrating on breathing evenly can also help you maintain your balance.

It is important to align your body correctly in this pose. As you perform the pose, keep your spine in a straight line and your head, shoulders and hips on the same plane.

If you feel any tension in your neck, do not turn your head up to look at your raised hand. Avoid Half Moon Pose if you are tired or have high blood pressure.

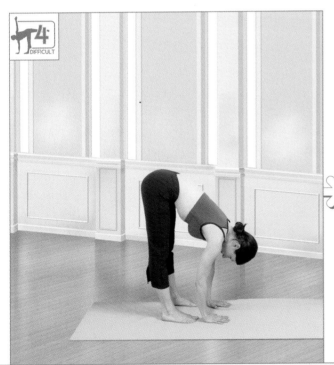

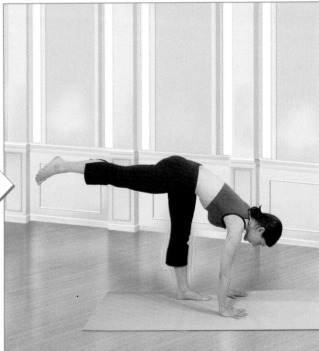

1 Begin in Mountain Pose. For information on Mountain Pose, see page 120.

2 Exhale as you bend forward from your hips, keeping your heels on the floor.

3 Place your palms on the floor in front of your feet. Your palms should be shoulder width apart.

• If you cannot place your palms on the floor, place your palms on blocks.

4 Shift your weight onto your left leg.

5 Exhale as you gradually lift and lengthen your right leg out behind you.

I find it difficult to balance in Half Moon Pose. What can I do?

You can use a wall to help maintain your balance in this pose. Stand with your left side to the wall. Perform the steps below, keeping the back of your head, shoulder blades, buttocks, raised heel and the back of your raised hand touching the wall as you hold the pose. In addition to keeping you balanced, the wall can help you align your body correctly.

Should I tighten my muscles while holding Half Moon Pose?

No. Tightening your muscles in Half Moon Pose will only make you unstable in the pose. Make sure you do not tense any part of your body as you hold the pose. Instead, focus on expanding and lengthening your body with each breath. Visualize your chest expanding as your arms stretch outward and your body lengthening from the crown of your head through to your raised foot.

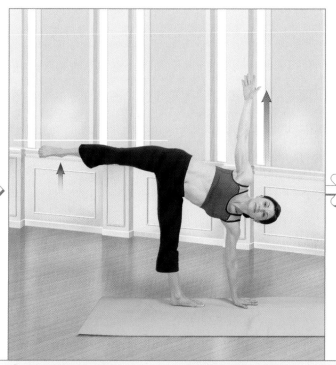

6 Exhale as you press your left heel into the floor and then lift your right palm off the floor as you turn your upper body to the right.

7 Inhale as you stretch your right arm up toward the ceiling, keeping your right shoulder back.

8 Continue to lift and lengthen your right leg until it is parallel to the floor.

9 Turn your head to gaze at your right hand, keeping your spine straight and your neck relaxed.

10 Hold the pose for 15 to 25 seconds.

11 To come out of the pose, exhale as you lower your right leg to the floor and lift your left palm off the floor. Then return to Mountain Pose.

12 Repeat steps 2 to 11 for your other side.

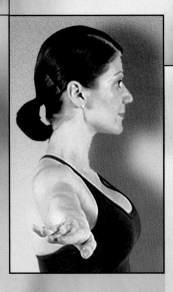

Chapter 9

Standing forward bends provide an excellent stretch for the back of your entire body and are useful for releasing tension. These poses can also help calm your mind and soothe your nervous system. Due to this calming effect, standing forward bends are especially beneficial when performed near the end of your yoga practice. This chapter offers several standing forward bends you can incorporate into your own practice.

Standing Forward Bends

In this Chapter...

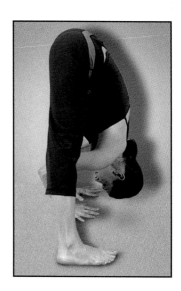

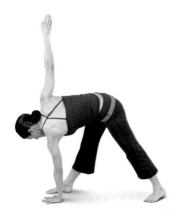

right angle pose

Right Angle Pose provides a deep stretch to your shoulders, arms, back and hamstrings. Stretching in this pose can relieve tension in your shoulders and upper back. This pose also helps to strengthen your wrists and legs.

While holding Right Angle Pose, try to picture your hands anchored to the wall. Then gently press your hands into the wall to lengthen your arms and back. You should also focus on keeping your shoulders and upper back wide. You may find it helpful to visualize your shoulders and upper back widening with each breath.

Resting your body weight on your legs in this pose strengthens your legs and reduces the weight your spine needs to support. As a result, your spine should feel light and relaxed. You may find this pose beneficial if you are pregnant, since positioning your body at a 90-degree angle will temporarily take the weight and pressure off your pelvis.

Use caution performing this pose if you have shoulder or back problems.

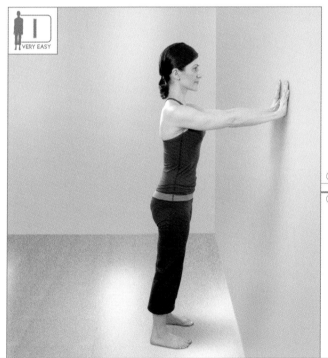

VERY EASY

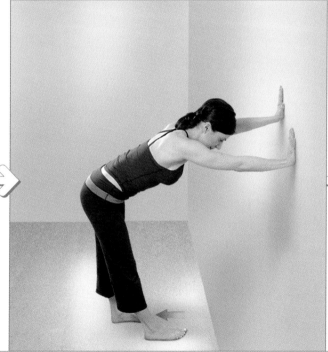

1 Stand in Mountain Pose facing a wall, with your body approximately one arm's length away from the wall. For information on Mountain Pose, see page 120.

2 Place your hands on the wall at shoulder height, with your fingers spread apart and your middle fingers pointing up.

3 Slowly walk backward.

4 Walk your hands down the wall with each step backward.

What should I do if my shoulders and back are rounded in this pose?

You should move your hands up the wall slightly so that your body forms an angle slightly greater than 90 degrees. Make sure you keep your arms and legs straight, but do not lock your elbows or knees.

Can I perform this pose if I have a wrist injury?

You can perform the pose, except you should place your forearms, rather than your hands, on the wall. Then walk backward until your feet are directly under your hips. As you inhale, press your forearms into the wall. As you exhale, drop your shoulders and upper back toward the floor.

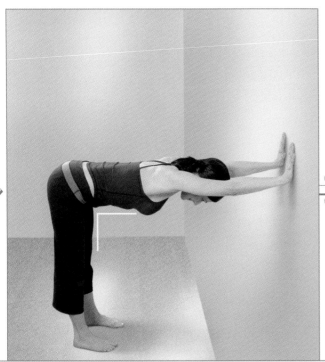

5 Bring your body to a 90-degree angle and position your feet hip to shoulder width apart.

• Make sure your back is flat, your legs are straight and your knees are not locked.

6 Gently press your hands into the wall as you lengthen through your arms and back.

• Make sure your head, neck and spine are in a straight line.

7 Hold the pose for 30 seconds to 1 minute and then return to Mountain Pose.

standing forward bend *(uttanasana)*

Standing Forward Bend stretches the entire back of your body, with an emphasis on stretching the back of your legs. This basic standing forward bend is often used as a resting pose between other standing poses.

Relaxing your head and neck toward the floor and lengthening your spine in this pose helps to release any tension in your upper body. Releasing tension in your upper body can help clear your mind, reduce fatigue and relieve stress.

If you find you cannot place your palms on the floor

in this pose, hang your arms loosely from your shoulders or bend your knees until you can touch the floor. Do not try to force your palms to the floor as you may strain your lower back. You should also try to keep your hips directly over your knees while performing the pose and avoid locking your knees.

Take caution performing Standing Forward Bend if you suffer from high blood pressure, lower back problems or headaches. If you become dizzy easily, be sure to come out of the pose very slowly.

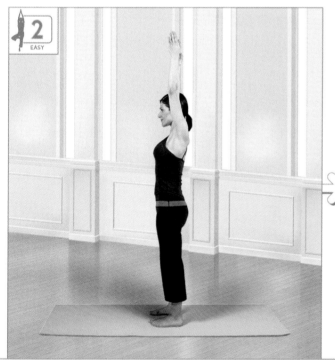

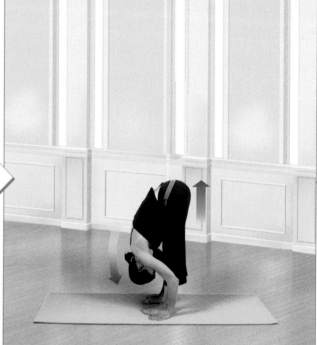

1 Begin in Mountain Pose. For information on Mountain Pose, see page 120.

2 Inhale as you stretch your arms above your head with your palms facing each other.

3 Stretch your entire body toward the ceiling, keeping your shoulders relaxed.

4 Exhale as you bend forward from your hips, keeping the soles of your feet pressed evenly into the floor.

5 Relax your head and neck toward the floor and lift your sitting bones toward the ceiling to lengthen your spine.

6 Place your palms on the floor on either side of your feet.

What should I do if the back of my legs feel strained while performing Standing Forward Bend?

If the back of your legs feel strained, you should keep your back flat, bend your knees and rest your hands on your thighs to perform the pose. As you gain flexibility, you can straighten your knees a little more each time you perform the pose. This modification is useful if you have high blood pressure, since your head stays above the level of your heart.

Can I perform Standing Forward Bend if I have lower back problems?

If you have lower back problems, you may want to perform a modified version of the pose. Perform the pose as described in the steps below, except rest your upper body on a table with your arms stretching forward across the table. You should still feel a stretch along the back of your legs while performing this modification. You can also perform Downward-Facing Dog Pose instead. For information on Downward-Facing Dog Pose, see page 188.

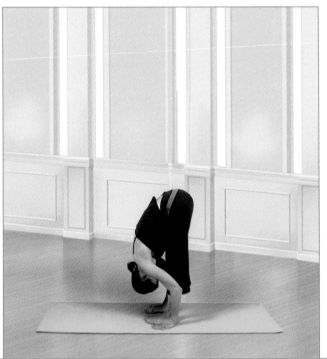

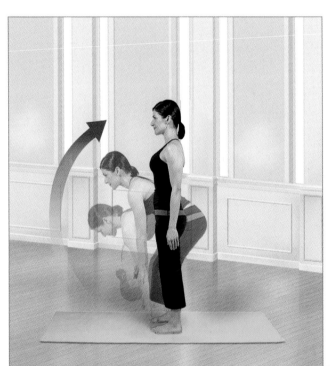

7 Exhale as you stretch the back of your legs and press your feet into the floor.

• Make sure your hips are directly above your knees and your knees are not locked.

• Visualize your torso lengthening toward the floor with each breath.

8 Hold the pose for 10 seconds to 1 minute.

Come Out of the Pose

1 Inhale as you bend your knees and slowly roll up to a standing position, pressing the soles of your feet evenly into the floor.

2 Return to Mountain Pose.

standing wide angle forward bend *(prasarita padottanasana)*

Standing Wide Angle Forward Bend provides an intense stretch to the back of your legs and also stretches your inner thighs. As with all forward bends, Standing Wide Angle Forward Bend can help release tension and improve circulation in your upper body. You may want to practice this pose after performing a series of standing poses to relieve fatigue.

As a general rule, you should stand with your feet approximately 3 feet apart when performing this pose. However, you can adjust your stance depending on your height. If you are tall, you should stand with your feet further apart. If you are short, you should stand with your feet closer together. Even after adjusting your stance, you may not be able to reach your palms down to the floor. In this case, you can rest each of your palms on a block or bend your knees.

Use caution performing this pose if you have high blood pressure or lower back problems. If you become dizzy easily, come out of the pose very slowly.

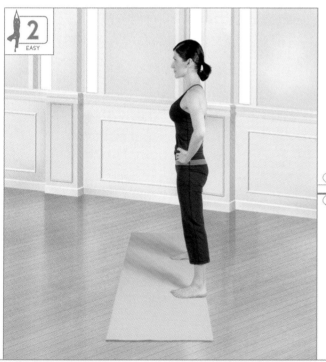

1 Begin in Mountain Pose. For information on Mountain Pose, see page 120.

2 Place your hands on your hips.

3 Step your right foot to the right 2 to 3 feet.

- Make sure your feet are parallel and your toes are pointing straight ahead.

4 Exhale as you bend forward from your hips, keeping your heels on the floor and your back flat.

5 Place your palms on the floor approximately shoulder width apart. Your arms should be straight.

6 Spread your fingers out, with your middle fingers pointing straight ahead.

7 Point the crown of your head toward the floor and tilt your sitting bones toward the ceiling to lengthen your spine.

How can I modify this pose if I have lower back problems?

If you have lower back problems, you can perform the pose using a wall for support. Begin in Mountain Pose facing a wall, about one arm's length away from the wall. Step your right foot to the right 2 to 3 feet and then place your palms on the wall. Bend forward from your hips, walking your hands down the wall until your upper body and legs form a 90-degree angle. Remember to keep your back straight and to lengthen your spine. This modification is also useful if you have high blood pressure.

How can I intensify the stretch in Standing Wide Angle Forward Bend?

Perform the pose as described below and then walk your hands back between your feet. As you walk your hands back, make sure you keep your hands shoulder width apart. This modification deepens the pose to intensify the stretch in the back of your legs and inner thighs.

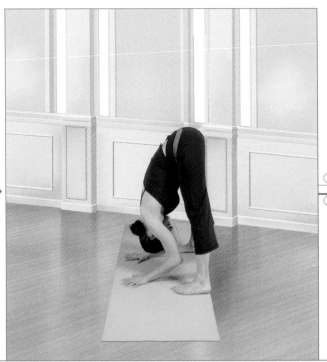

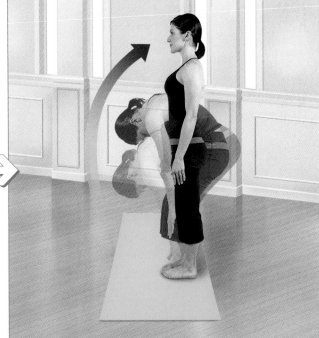

8 Exhale as you bend your elbows and bring your chest toward the space between your thighs.

9 Relax your head and neck toward the floor and feel your spine lengthening.

• Make sure your knees are not locked.

• Visualize the back of your legs and your inner thighs stretching with each breath.

10 Hold the pose for 30 seconds to 1 minute.

11 To come out of the pose, bring your feet together. Inhale as you bend your knees and slowly roll up to a standing position. Then return to Mountain Pose.

standing forward
bend twist

Standing Forward Bend Twist provides an intense stretch to the back of your legs and to your inner thighs, while twisting your spine. This pose is beneficial for toning your abdominal muscles, releasing tension in your upper body and improving your circulation.

As you perform Standing Forward Bend Twist, focus on moving deeper into the twist with each exhalation. The position of your arms in this pose opens your chest to increase your capacity for deep breathing. If you find looking up at your raised hand strains your neck, you can look at the floor instead.

Before performing Standing Forward Bend Twist, you should feel comfortable performing Standing Wide Angle Forward Bend, which is a more basic variation of this pose. Practicing Standing Wide Angle Forward Bend can help you develop the balance and flexibility you need to perform this pose.

Take caution performing Standing Forward Bend Twist if you suffer from high blood pressure, lower back problems or headaches.

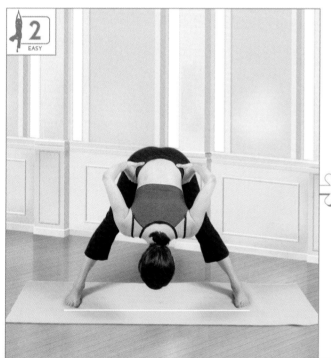

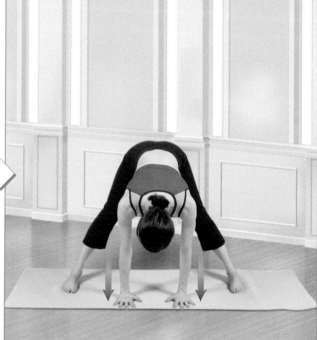

1 Begin in Mountain Pose. For information on Mountain Pose, see page 120.

2 Step your right foot to the right 2 to 3 feet.

• Make sure your feet are parallel and your toes are pointing straight ahead.

3 Exhale as you bend forward from your hips, keeping your heels on the floor and your back flat.

4 Place your palms on the floor in front of you. Your arms should be straight and your elbows should not be locked.

5 Point the crown of your head toward the floor and tilt your sitting bones toward the ceiling to lengthen your spine.

• Make sure your head, neck and spine are in a straight line.

How do I know if the width of my stance is correct in this pose?

As a general rule, you should stand with your feet 2 to 3 feet apart in this pose. However, you may need to adjust your stance if you are tall. Standing with your feet further than 3 feet apart may help you reach your palms to the floor.

What should I do if I cannot reach my palms to the floor?

If you cannot reach your palms down to the floor, you can rest each of your palms on a block or bend your knees slightly.

I find I get dizzy when I perform this pose. What should I do?

Make sure you breathe evenly as you perform the twist and come out of the pose very slowly. Avoid this pose if dizziness continues to be a problem.

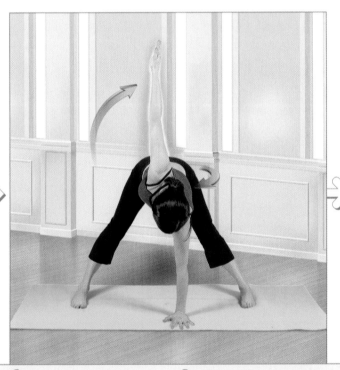

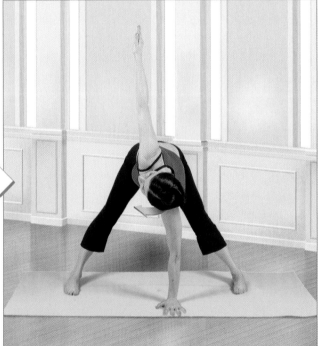

6 Press your left hand into the floor.

7 Inhale as you raise your right arm and point your fingers toward the ceiling.

8 Twist your torso to the right.

9 Turn your head and look up at your right hand.

10 Hold the pose for 15 to 30 seconds.

11 Repeat steps 6 to 10 for your other side.

12 To come out of the pose, release the twist and bring your feet together. Bend your knees and inhale as you slowly roll up to a standing position.

side angle twist *(parivrtta parsvakonasana)*

Side Angle Twist, also called Reverse Right Angle, is an advanced pose that stretches your legs, spine and the sides of your body. The twist in this pose stimulates your abdominal organs, which helps to aid digestion. Side Angle Twist is also useful for improving your balance and strengthening your legs and torso.

While performing Side Angle Twist, make sure you keep your back flat and your spine lengthened. You should also make sure you keep your arms straight.

The position of your arms in this pose allows your chest to open more, which can increase your capacity for deep breathing. Since the twist in this pose is intense, be careful not to move deeper into the pose than is comfortable for you.

You should use caution performing Side Angle Twist if you have had an injury to your back or spine or if you have high blood pressure. You should also avoid this pose if you have a headache.

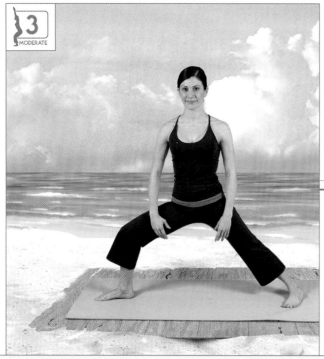

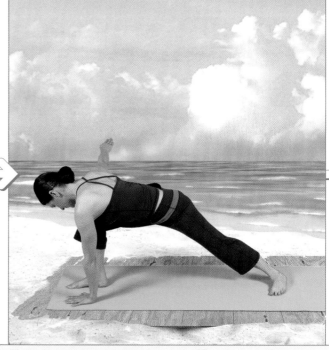

1 Begin in Mountain Pose. For information on Mountain Pose, see page 120.

2 Step your right foot to the right approximately 3 feet.

3 Turn your left foot in 45 degrees and then turn your right foot out 90 degrees.

4 Bend your right knee until it is over your right ankle.

5 Turn your torso to face the same direction as your right knee.

6 Raise your arms up to shoulder height, with your palms facing down. Your shoulders should be down and relaxed.

7 Exhale as you bend forward from your hips.

8 Place your left palm or fingertips on the floor near the inside of your right foot.

What can I do if I have difficulty maintaining my balance?

To help maintain your balance, begin in Lunge Pose with your left knee on the floor. For information on Lunge Pose, see page 180. Then perform steps 6 to 12 below and repeat for your other side. Once you become comfortable with this modification, try the pose from the standing position. This modification is also useful if you have high blood pressure and must avoid a standing forward bend.

What should I do if my palm cannot reach the floor?

If your palm cannot reach the floor in this pose, you can position a block on the inside of your foot and place your palm on the block.

How can I deepen this pose?

To deepen the pose, place your palm or fingertips on the floor on the outside of your foot. This modification provides a more intense twist to your torso and spine.

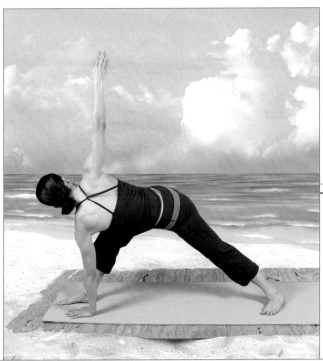

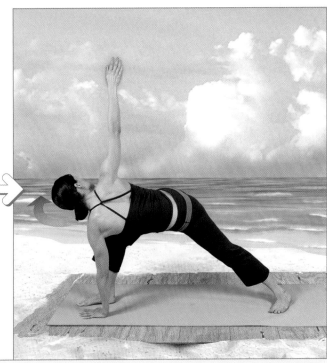

9 Twist to the right and stretch your right arm up toward the ceiling. Your arm should be straight, but your elbow should not be locked.

10 Turn your head to look up at your right hand.

11 Press through the crown of your head to lengthen your spine.

12 Hold the pose for 15 to 30 seconds.

13 To come out of the pose, bring your right arm down and release the twist in your torso. Then return to Mountain Pose.

14 Repeat steps 2 to 13 for your other side.

pyramid pose *(parsvottanasana)*

Pyramid Pose is a standing forward bend that provides an intense stretch to the back of your legs, while lengthening and releasing your spine. Regular practice of Pyramid Pose can relieve tension in your neck and shoulders, strengthen your legs, increase the flexibility of your hips and improve your balance.

Your lower body, from your waist down, forms the foundation of the pose and must be stable before you bend forward. You can adjust the position of your feet until your lower body feels stable and grounded.

Bending forward in the pose may cause you to lift your back heel off the floor. You should focus on keeping your back heel in contact with the floor to maintain stability.

You will feel an intense stretch in your front leg as you bend forward, which may cause you to hyperextend or lock your knee. Make sure you keep your front knee soft, but not bent.

Avoid performing Pyramid Pose if you have high blood pressure or heart problems.

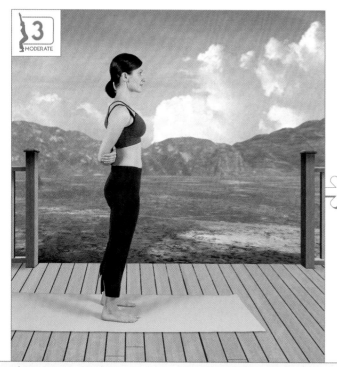

3 MODERATE

1 Begin in Mountain Pose. For information on Mountain Pose, see page 120.

2 Bend your elbows and move your forearms behind your back.

3 Clasp your elbows or wrists behind your back.

4 Exhale as you step your right foot forward approximately 3 feet.

5 Turn your left foot out 45 degrees and press the soles of your feet firmly into the floor.

• If you do not feel stable, adjust the position of your feet until you do.

I do not feel stable in Pyramid Pose. What can I do?

If you do not feel stable while performing Pyramid Pose, you can place your palms on the floor on either side of your front foot, instead of folding your arms behind your back. If you cannot reach the floor, position blocks on either side of your front foot and place your palms on the blocks. You should still keep your back heel in contact with the floor while performing either of these modified versions of the pose.

How can I make Pyramid Pose more challenging?

If you want to make Pyramid Pose more challenging, you can perform the pose with your hands positioned behind your back in Reverse Prayer Pose. Positioning your hands in Reverse Prayer Pose will increase the stretch in your chest and shoulders, as well as challenge your ability to maintain your balance. For information on Reverse Prayer Pose, see page 48.

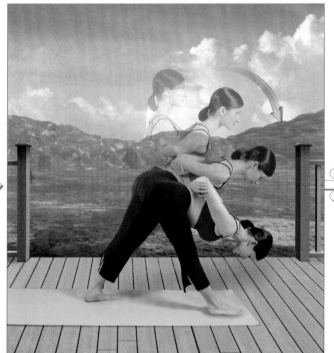

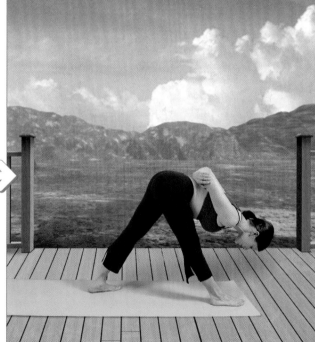

6 Exhale as you bend forward from your hips over your right leg, keeping your back flat and your left heel in contact with the floor.

• As you bend forward, you will feel a stretch in the back of your right leg.

7 Allow your spine to lengthen as you relax your head and neck toward the floor.

8 Hold the pose for 15 to 30 seconds.

9 To come out of the pose, press your right foot into the floor and then slowly roll up, keeping your left heel in contact with the floor. Then return to Mountain Pose.

10 Repeat steps 2 to 9 for your other side.

triangle twist *(parivrtta trikonasana)*

Triangle Twist is an advanced pose that provides an intense stretch to your legs and the sides of your body. You can also use this pose to strengthen your legs, increase the flexibility of your hips, relieve tension in your back and improve your balance.

While performing Triangle Twist, make sure you keep your back flat and your spine lengthened. You should also make sure you keep your arms straight. The position of your arms in this pose allows your chest to open more, which can increase your capacity for deep breathing.

If you find Triangle Twist difficult, you may need to place your palm on a block if you cannot reach down to the floor. You may also need to come out of the twist slightly if your knee feels strained.

Always use caution performing this pose if you have a back or spine injury or high blood pressure. You should avoid this pose if you have a headache.

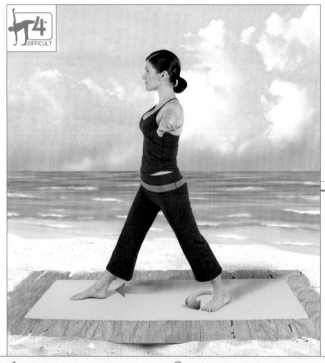

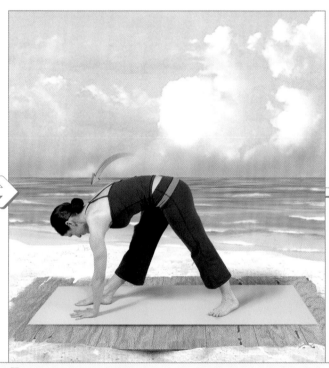

1 Begin in Mountain Pose. For information on Mountain Pose, see page 120.

2 Step your right foot forward approximately 3 feet.

3 Turn your left foot out 45 degrees and press the soles of your feet into the floor.

4 Raise your arms up to shoulder height, with your palms facing down. Your shoulders should be down and relaxed.

5 Exhale as you bend forward from your hips over your right leg, keeping your back flat and your left heel in contact with the floor.

• Make sure both your legs are straight, but your knees are not locked.

6 Place your left palm or fingertips on the floor near the inside of your right foot.

How can I modify this pose if I have stiff shoulders?

Instead of stretching your upper arm toward the ceiling, rest your arm on your side. This modification is also useful if your upper arm feels strained or uncomfortable in the pose.

I have neck problems and cannot look up at my raised hand. Can I still perform the pose?

Yes. You can modify the pose by looking straight ahead or down at the floor instead of looking up at your raised hand.

How can I deepen this pose?

To deepen the pose, place your palm or fingertips on the floor on the outside of your foot. This modification provides a more intense twist to your torso and spine.

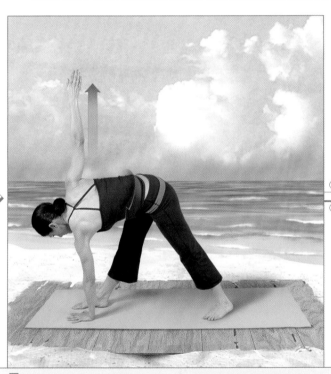

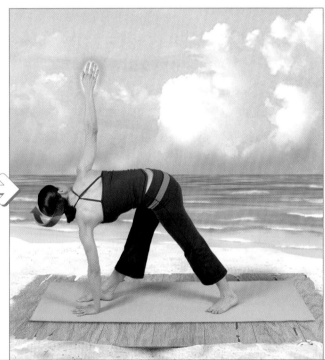

7 Stretch your right arm up toward the ceiling. Your arm should be straight, but your elbow should not be locked.

• Your torso should turn to face your right leg.

8 Turn your head to look up at your right hand.

9 Press through the crown of your head to lengthen your spine.

10 Hold the pose for 15 to 30 seconds. Then exhale, bring your right arm down and release the twist in your torso. Then return to Mountain Pose.

11 Repeat steps 2 to 10 for your other side.

standing yoga
mudra pose *(dandayamana yoga mudra)*

Standing Yoga Mudra Pose provides an intense stretch to your shoulders. This pose also stretches your upper back and legs, while helping to increase the flexibility of your spine and hips.

You can perform Standing Yoga Mudra Pose to help clear your mind, center your thoughts and become more aware of your feelings.

As you move into the pose, try to keep your palms together to maintain the intensity of the stretch in your shoulders. Stretching your arms back and up in this

pose can help correct a rounded back and shoulders.

While holding the pose, you may find the stretch in the back of your legs too intense. Try standing with your feet further apart to reduce the strain. With regular practice of this pose, you should eventually be able to bring your legs closer together.

You should use caution performing this pose if you have high blood pressure or an injury to your neck, shoulders, back or legs.

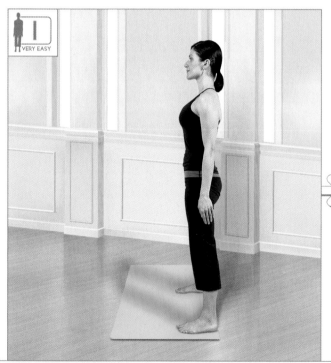

VERY EASY

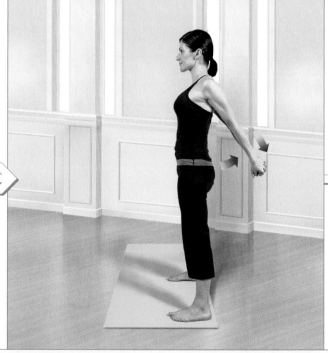

1 Begin in Mountain Pose. For information on Mountain Pose, see page 120.

2 Step your right foot to the right to position your feet slightly wider than hip width apart.

• Your feet should be parallel and your toes should be pointing forward.

3 Interlace your fingers behind your back.

4 Press your hands down away from your shoulders to lengthen your arms.

• Feel your shoulder blades come together as your chest opens.

I have difficulty interlacing my fingers behind my back. What can I do?

If you have difficulty interlacing your fingers behind your back, you can hold a strap with your hands as close together on the strap as is comfortable for you. Holding a strap puts less strain on your shoulders because your hands can be further apart.

How can I make this pose more challenging?

You can perform Yoga Mudra Warrior Pose, which is a more difficult version of Standing Yoga Mudra Pose. To perform Yoga Mudra Warrior Pose, begin in Warrior I Pose, as shown on page 128, with your front knee bent at a 90-degree angle. Then interlace your fingers behind your back and lean your torso forward over your bent leg, raising your arms up behind you. Only raise your arms as far as is comfortable for you.

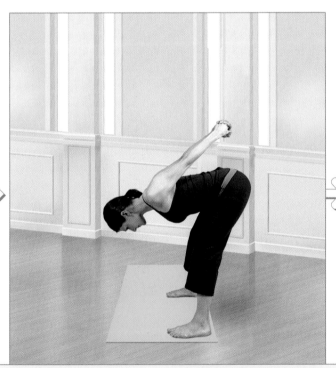

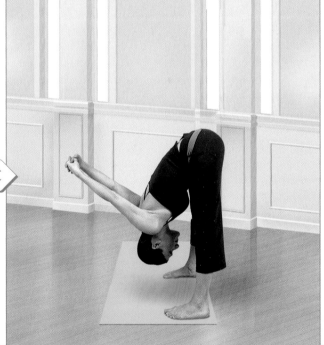

5 Exhale as you bend forward from your hips.

• Allow your arms to lift up behind you.

6 Bend your knees slightly to lessen the strain in your lower back and legs.

7 Raise your arms behind you as far as is comfortable for you.

• Your head moves further toward the floor as your arms move away from your body.

8 Hold the pose for 30 seconds to 1 minute.

9 To come out of the pose, press out through your hands and keep your back flat as you lift your torso up.

rag doll pose

Rag Doll Pose is beneficial for relieving tension in your head, neck, shoulders and lower back. This pose is also useful for lengthening your spine and increasing the flexibility in the back of your legs. You may want to perform Rag Doll Pose to rest after performing more strenuous standing poses, such as Triangle Pose.

Rag Doll Pose is a more relaxed variation of Standing Forward Bend, which is shown on page 154. You may want to perform Rag Doll Pose to prepare for Standing Forward Bend.

While performing Rag Doll Pose, your upper body should hang loose and relaxed like a rag doll. If you have a weak lower back, make sure you bend your knees and roll up one vertebra at a time as you come out of the pose. You should also come out of the pose slowly if you become dizzy easily.

You should use caution performing Rag Doll Pose if you have a back injury, high blood pressure or an eye problem, such as glaucoma.

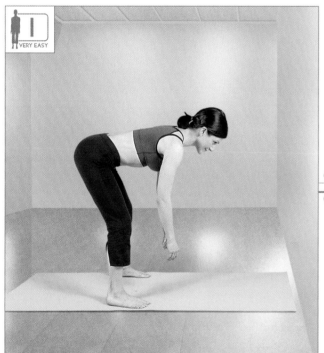

VERY EASY

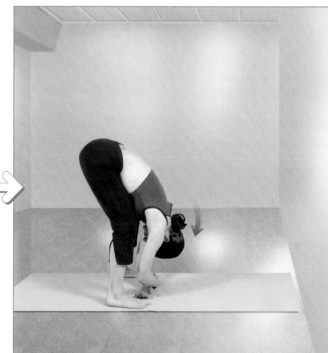

1 Begin in Mountain Pose. For information on Mountain Pose, see page 120.

2 Step your right foot to the right 2 to 3 feet.

3 Exhale as you bend forward from your hips, keeping the soles of your feet pressed evenly into the floor.

4 Bend your knees slightly.

5 Relax your head and neck toward the floor to lengthen your spine.

6 Let your arms dangle toward the floor.

• Visualize yourself as a rag doll, hanging limp and relaxed.

What can I do to relax my upper body and neck more in Rag Doll Pose?

Perform the pose as described below, except sway your upper body from side to side. To further relax your neck, gently nod your head up and down while performing the pose. You can also gently shake your head from side to side.

Can I vary the position of my arms in this pose?

Yes. Instead of allowing your arms to dangle toward the floor, you can fold your arms so that each elbow rests in the palm of your opposite hand. Then let your elbows hang down toward the floor as you hold the pose.

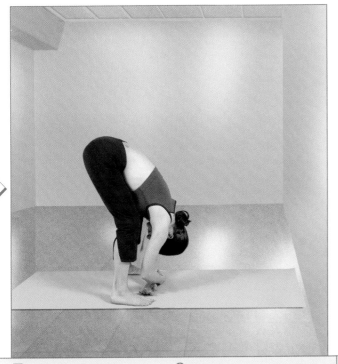

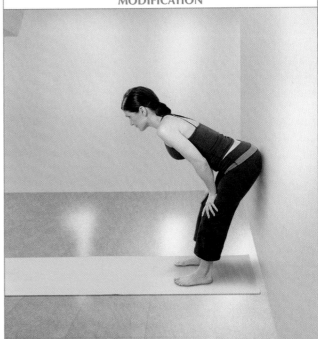

MODIFICATION

7 Hold the pose for 10 to 30 seconds. With each exhalation, allow yourself to relax a little more into the pose.

8 To come out of the pose, inhale as you bend your knees and slowly roll up to a standing position, pressing the soles of your feet evenly into the floor. Then return to Mountain Pose.

• You can use a wall for support and rest your hands on your thighs. This modification is beneficial if you have high blood pressure.

1 Lean back against a wall, allowing the wall to support your weight as you bend forward.

2 Rest your hands on your thighs. Keep your knees relaxed, your back flat and your head above your heart.

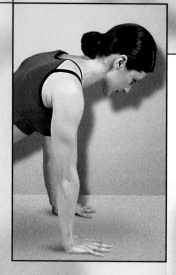

Chapter 10

Table poses are beneficial for aligning your spine, as well as stretching and strengthening your arms and legs. In table poses, you usually support the weight of your body on your hands and knees or feet, which can help strengthen your bones. Building strong bones can prevent a bone disease that causes your bones to become fragile and prone to breakage. This chapter demonstrates a variety of table poses.

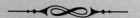

Table Poses

In this Chapter...

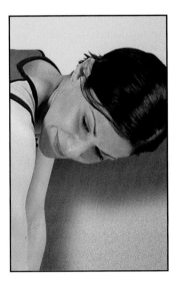

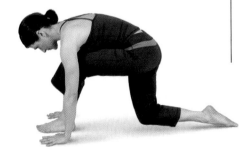

table pose

Table Pose is beneficial for correctly aligning your spine. You can also use this pose as a transition between poses or as a starting position for another pose. For example, you can use Table Pose as a transition to Downward-Facing Dog Pose. For information on Downward-Facing Dog Pose, see page 188.

By supporting the weight of your body with your hands and knees, this pose can help strengthen your bones. Building strong bones can help prevent osteoporosis—a bone disease that causes your bones to deteriorate, becoming fragile and prone to breaks.

While performing Table Pose, make sure you keep your head aligned with your spine. It is common for beginners to make the mistake of dropping their heads down while in Table Pose.

If you feel pressure on your knees in this pose, try placing a folded towel or blanket under them to relieve the strain. You should avoid Table Pose if you have knee problems or wrist problems, such as Carpal Tunnel Syndrome.

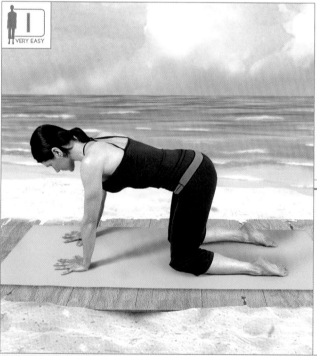

VERY EASY

1 Position yourself on your hands and knees, with your knees and feet hip width apart.

- Your knees should be directly under your hips and the top of your feet should be on the floor.

- Your wrists should be directly under your shoulders and your palms should be on the floor.

2 Spread your fingers out, with your middle fingers pointing forward.

3 Press your hands into the floor and relax your shoulders down. Your arms should be straight, but your elbows should not be locked.

- Make sure your back is flat and your head is aligned with your spine.

4 Extend your tailbone behind you and the crown of your head in front of you to lengthen your spine.

5 Hold the pose for 20 seconds to 1 minute.

side cat stretch

Side Cat Stretch is a good warm-up pose that stretches the sides of your body and opens your rib cage. If you have a back or hip problem that prevents you from sitting comfortably on the floor, you may want to use this pose as an alternative to seated poses that stretch the sides of your body.

While performing Side Cat Stretch, you should feel one side of your body lengthen as the other side squeezes. On the lengthened side of your body, focus on feeling the stretch in your waist, hip, shoulder and neck.

As you move your body in this pose, remember to keep your hips over your knees and to move your hips from side to side, not forward and backward. Also, make sure your head follows the movement of your body rather than leading the movement.

Use caution performing this pose if you have wrist problems, such as Carpal Tunnel Syndrome, or a knee injury.

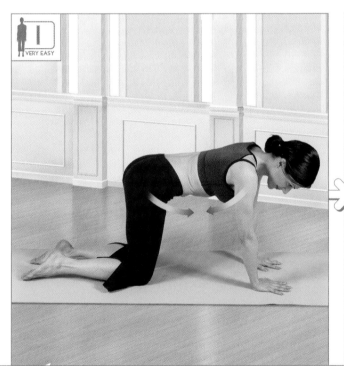

VERY EASY

1 Begin in Table Pose. For information on Table Pose, see page 172.

- Your back should be flat and your head should be in line with your spine.

2 Move your right shoulder and right hip toward each other.

- Your body should create a C shape.

3 Turn your head to look over your right shoulder toward your hip.

4 Hold the pose for 5 to 30 seconds and then return to Table Pose.

5 Repeat for your other side.

6 Repeat steps 2 to 5 six times.

cat stretch *(marjarasana)*

Cat Stretch improves the flexibility of your spine and the circulation in your torso. While stretching your shoulders, back and hips, this stretch may also help improve many bodily functions, such as digestion and elimination. You may want to perform Cat Stretch as a warm-up pose or after more strenuous poses to help release tension from your body.

Cat Stretch allows you to practice coordinating your movements with your breath. Exhale as you round and lift your upper back and inhale as you gently arch your lower back. Remember to keep the movements

in Cat Stretch smooth and fluid.

You should use your entire spine to perform this stretch, making sure the back of your neck and your lower back are not compressed when you curl your spine. Feel your spine lengthen in each direction as your tailbone moves away from the crown of your head. As you round and lift your upper back, keep your shoulders relaxed down.

You should use caution performing Cat Stretch if you have back, wrist or knee problems.

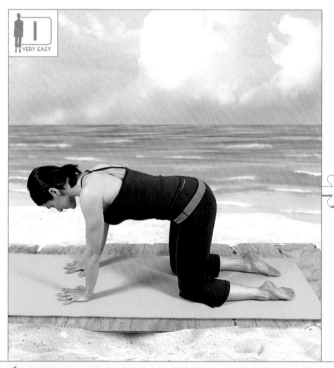

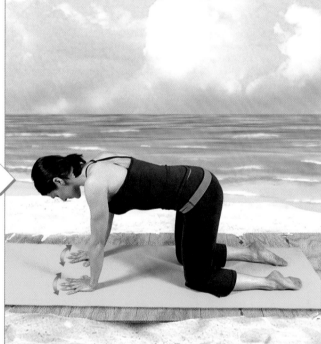

1 Begin in Table Pose. For information on Table Pose, see page 172.

- Make sure your wrists are below your shoulders and your knees are below your hips.

- Make sure your arms are straight, but your elbows are not locked.

2 Spread your fingers out, with your middle fingers pointing straight ahead.

3 Lengthen your spine, keeping your head, neck and spine in a straight line.

How can I modify the stretch if I have wrist problems?

If you have wrist problems, you can make your hands into fists and place your knuckles, instead of your palms, on the floor as you perform Cat Stretch. You can also perform the stretch with your wrists supported. To support your wrists, place a rolled up towel under your wrists and allow your fingers to rest on the floor.

My knees feel sore when I perform Cat Stretch. What can I do?

You can place a folded blanket under your knees. If you cannot rest on your knees at all, you can perform Cat Stretch sitting in Easy Pose, which is shown on page 74. Exhale as you round your back and tuck your chin toward your chest. Then inhale as you press your sitting bones into the floor, lift your chest up and point the crown of your head toward the ceiling.

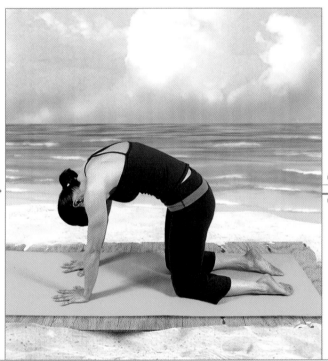

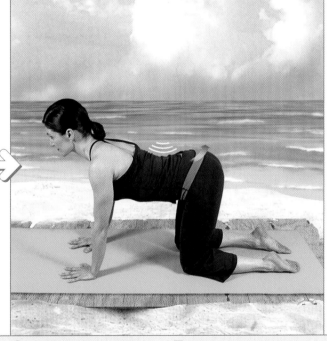

4 Supporting the weight of your body evenly on your hands and knees, exhale as you tuck your tailbone under you and round and lift your upper back toward the ceiling.

5 Tuck your chin toward your chest.

• Visualize yourself as a cat stretching after waking up from a nap.

6 Inhale as you curl your tailbone up toward the ceiling so your stomach moves toward the floor and your lower back gently arches.

7 Point the crown of your head toward the ceiling and gaze straight ahead.

8 Repeat steps 4 to 7 three to ten times.

extended cat stretch

Extended Cat Stretch is a great pose for stretching and warming up your spine. This pose is also beneficial for stretching your legs and neck. By supporting the weight of your body in this pose with your hands and knees, you strengthen your wrists and arms and help build strong bones. If you are feeling sluggish, you can perform Extended Cat Stretch to help awaken and energize your mind.

As you bring your forehead toward your knee in Extended Cat Stretch, make sure you do not strain your neck. You should only move your forehead as close to your knee as is comfortable for you.

Use caution performing Extended Cat Stretch if you have wrist problems, such as Carpal Tunnel Syndrome. If you find that your wrists need extra support when performing the stretch, you can place a rolled up towel under your wrists, allowing your fingers to rest on the floor. You should also be careful performing this pose if you have a knee injury.

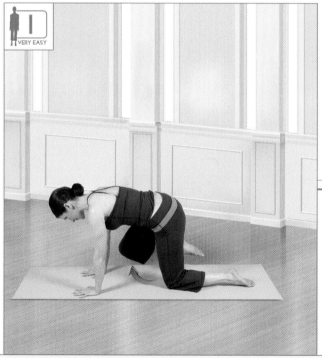

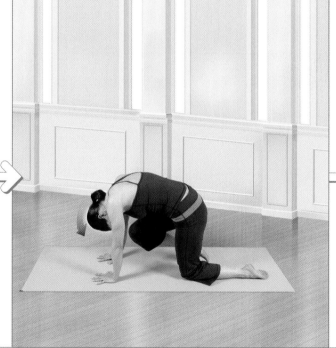

1 Begin in Table Pose. For information on Table Pose, see page 172.

2 Exhale as you bring your right knee off the floor and under your body.

3 Tuck your forehead down.

• Your forehead and right knee should move toward each other.

What should I do if my knees are uncomfortable in this pose?

If you feel pressure on your knees in this pose, place a folded towel or blanket under your knees before you begin. This makes the pose more comfortable, protecting your supporting knee from any stress you may experience as you raise your other leg.

How can I ensure my pelvis is stable in this pose?

It is important to make sure your pelvis is stable and your hips are even and facing the floor in this pose. To help stabilize your pelvis, try to focus on pulling your abdominal muscles toward your spine. You should also make sure you do not lean into your supporting leg.

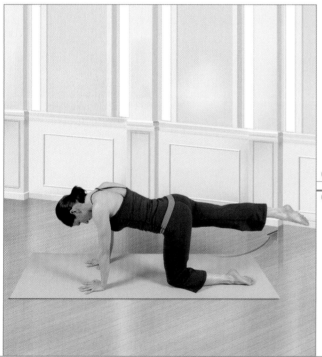

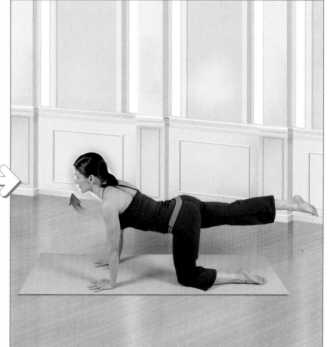

4 Inhale as you extend your right leg behind you.

- Make sure both your hips are facing the floor and your pelvis is stable.

5 Point the toes of your right foot behind you and stretch through your toes.

6 Lift your head and look forward.

- Feel your body lengthening from the crown of your head to the tips of your toes.

7 Repeat steps 2 to 6 three to six times and then return to Table Pose.

8 Repeat steps 2 to 7 for your other side.

table balancing pose

Table Balancing Pose is an energizing pose that improves your balance and strengthens your entire body. This pose also stretches your arms and legs and helps to align your spine.

By supporting the weight of your body on your hands and knees, Table Balancing Pose helps strengthen your bones. Building strong bones can prevent osteoporosis—a bone disease that causes your bones to deteriorate, becoming fragile and prone to breaks.

While performing this pose, you should keep your hips even and facing the floor. To keep your hips even, make sure you do not lean into your leg that remains on the floor. You should also pull your abdominal muscles toward your spine to maintain stability in your pelvis. As you hold the pose, try to visualize your breath energizing your body and mind.

You should use caution performing Table Balancing Pose if you have problems with your wrists, such as Carpal Tunnel Syndrome, or a knee injury.

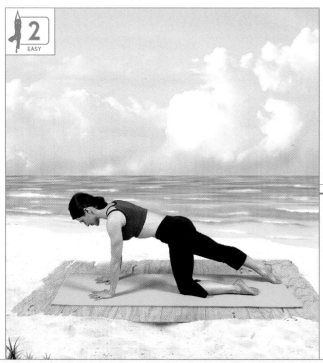

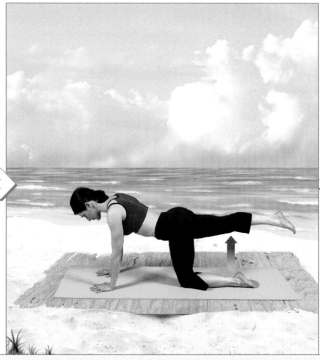

1 Begin in Table Pose. For information on Table Pose, see page 172.

2 Extend your right leg behind you, keeping the top of your right foot on the floor.

3 Lift your right leg to hip height.

• Make sure your hips are even and facing the floor.

I have difficulty balancing in this pose. What can I do?

You can keep both hands on the floor when you raise your leg. Once you feel comfortable balancing with both hands on the floor and your leg raised, you can try lifting your arm.

You can also perform the pose as described in the steps below, except place the sole of the foot of your raised leg against a wall for support. This modification helps you build the strength needed to hold the pose on your own.

What should I do if my supporting knee is uncomfortable in this pose?

If you feel pressure on your supporting knee in this pose, you can place a folded towel or blanket under your knee to make the pose more comfortable.

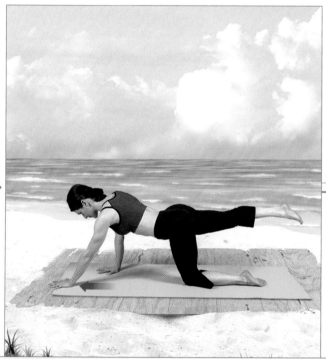

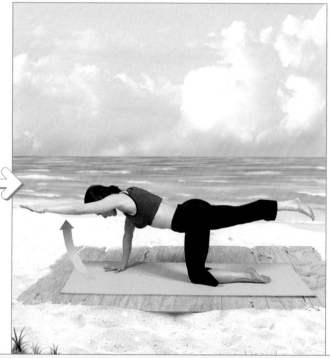

4 Extend your left arm in front of you, keeping your left palm on the floor.

• Your back should be flat and your head should be in line with your spine.

5 Lift your left arm to shoulder height.

6 Press out through the fingertips of your left hand, the crown of your head and the toes of your right foot.

7 Hold the pose for 30 seconds to 1 minute and then return to Table Pose.

8 Repeat steps 2 to 7 for your other side.

lunge pose *(ashwa sanchalanasana)*

Lunge Pose stretches your legs and groin, with an emphasis on stretching the front of your thighs. This pose also lengthens your spine and helps to open your chest and hips.

Increasing the flexibility of your hips in Lunge Pose can help you sit more comfortably in poses, such as Easy Pose and Bound Angle Pose. Lunge Pose can also make performing back bends easier by increasing the flexibility in the front of your thighs. Lunge Pose is often performed as part of Sun Salutation. For

information on Sun Salutation, see page 262.

To avoid rounding your lower back in Lunge Pose, make sure that you keep your back flat and your spine lengthened. Try to visualize the lengthening of your spine and the lifting of your torso as you inhale, and the sinking of your hips as you exhale.

If you feel pressure on your back knee in this pose, place a blanket under your knee to make the pose more comfortable. Always use caution performing Lunge Pose if you have knee or hip problems.

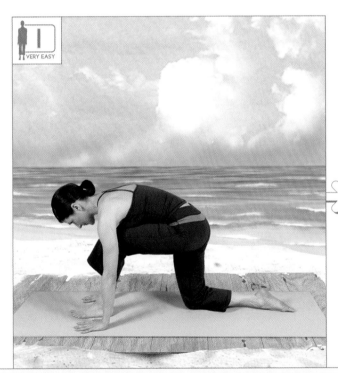

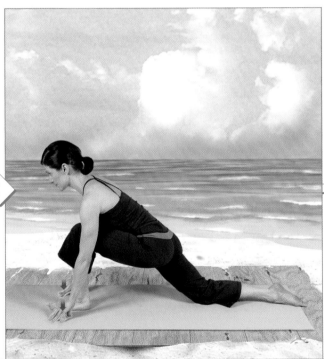

1 Begin in Table Pose. For information on Table Pose, see page 172.

2 Step your left foot forward and place your foot between your hands.

• Your left knee should be directly over your left ankle and both hips should be facing forward.

3 Press your fingers or palms into the floor, lift your torso upward and relax your shoulders back and down.

• Feel the stretch in the front of your right thigh and feel your right hip gently moving forward and down.

4 Tuck your tailbone under to lengthen your spine.

What should I do if my hands cannot reach the floor?

If your hands cannot reach the floor in this pose, you can place your palms on blocks to help lift your torso upward.

Can I make Lunge Pose more challenging for my legs?

To work your leg muscles more, lift your torso up and rest your palms on your front thigh. Then press your palms into your thigh to lift your torso upward. Remember to keep your shoulders relaxed back and down.

Can I use Lunge Pose to improve my balance?

While holding the pose, raise your arms above your head, with your palms facing each other. Then bring your palms together, keeping your arms stretched up toward the ceiling and your shoulders relaxed down. Point the crown of your head toward the ceiling and gaze straight ahead. This modification helps to improve your balance, open your chest and stretch your arms and shoulders.

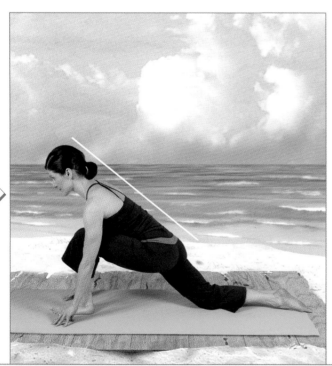

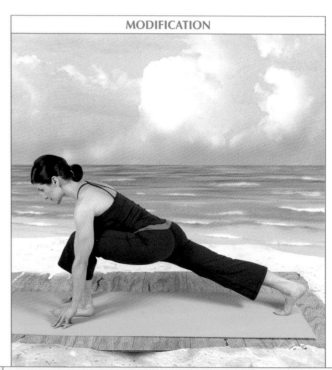

MODIFICATION

5 Elongate the back of your neck and keep your head in alignment with your spine. Your head should not drop forward toward your chest.

6 Hold the pose for 30 seconds to 1 minute and then return to Table Pose.

7 Repeat steps 2 to 6 for your other side.

• You can intensify the stretch of Lunge Pose by raising your back knee off the floor.

1 Perform Lunge Pose, except curl the toes of your right foot under and straighten your right leg. Then move the back of your right leg toward the ceiling as you extend your right heel toward the floor.

thread the needle pose

Thread the Needle Pose is an asymmetrical pose that stretches your shoulders and upper back. This pose is also useful for stretching your neck and arms. You may find performing this pose gives you a feeling of contentment when you are upset or distressed.

This pose is called Thread the Needle Pose because you thread one arm under the other. By threading one arm under your other arm and resting your shoulder and ear on the floor, this pose provides a gentle twist to your spine.

You can practice Thread the Needle Pose to prepare for performing inverted poses, such as Shoulderstand and Plow Pose.

If you feel pressure on your knees in this pose, you can place a folded towel or blanket under your knees to make the pose more comfortable. Make sure you use caution performing this pose if you have problems with your neck, shoulders or knees.

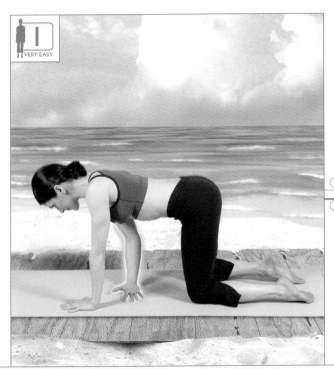

VERY EASY

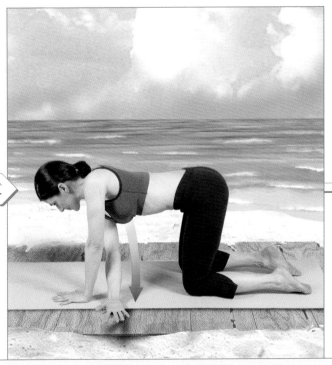

1 Begin in Table Pose. For information on Table Pose, see page 172.

2 Place your right hand under your body, with your palm facing up.

3 Exhale as you slide your right arm further under your body.

• Your right hand should extend past the left side of your body, between your left hand and left knee.

What should I do if my shoulder and ear do not reach the floor in this pose?

You can place a folded towel or blanket under your shoulder and head for support if you cannot reach your shoulder and ear to the floor. This modification is also useful if your shoulder and ear are uncomfortable on the floor.

How can I deepen Thread the Needle Pose?

Perform the pose as described in the steps below, except after holding the pose, inhale and stretch your left arm up toward the ceiling. Stretching your arm up helps to open your chest. You can also deepen the pose by extending your left leg on a diagonal to the side with the sole of your left foot on the floor. Then stretch your left arm up toward the ceiling. Repeat these modifications for your other side.

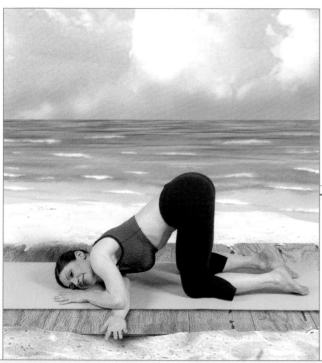

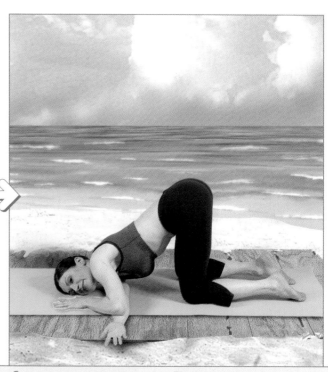

4 Lower your right shoulder and right ear to the floor.

• Make sure you keep your left arm relaxed as you rest your right arm and hand on the floor.

5 Hold the pose for 30 seconds to 1 minute.

6 To come out of the pose, press your left hand into the floor to lift your body up. Then return to Table Pose.

7 Repeat steps 2 to 6 for your other side.

plank pose

Plank Pose strengthens your arms, wrists and upper body. This pose also tones your abdominal muscles and helps to lengthen your spine. By supporting the weight of your body with your arms, this pose can strengthen your bones. Building strong bones can help prevent osteoporosis—a bone disease that causes your bones to deteriorate, becoming fragile and prone to breaks.

Plank Pose is commonly performed as part of Sun Salutation. For information on Sun Salutation, see page 262.

Make sure you do not raise your buttocks up too high or drop your pelvis or chest toward the floor. Your body should form a straight line from your head to your heels. You can tighten your abdominal muscles to help keep your body in a straight line. As you maintain this straight line, focus on lengthening your spine. You should also concentrate on moving your breath through your entire body to release any tension.

You should avoid Plank Pose if you have wrist problems, such as Carpal Tunnel Syndrome.

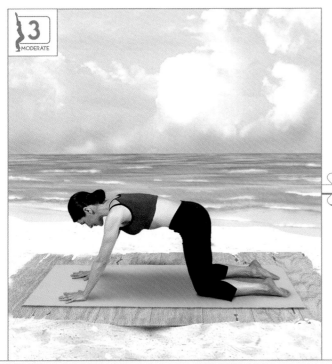

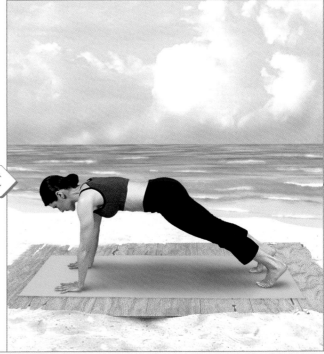

1 Begin in Table Pose. For information on Table Pose, see page 172.

2 Move your hands forward approximately 6 inches.

3 Press your hands into the floor and then curl your toes under.

4 Inhale as you straighten your legs to position yourself on your hands and feet.

- You may need to adjust the position of your hands so your body forms a straight line.

- Keep your wrists directly under your shoulders. Your arms should be straight, but your elbows should not be locked.

I find Plank Pose difficult to hold. What can I do?

If you find the pose too difficult to hold, you can lower your knees to the floor. With your knees on the floor, rest the top of your feet on the floor and make sure your upper body and thighs form a straight line from your knees to your shoulders. This modification is especially useful if your arms are not strong enough to support your body or if your upper body is weak or injured.

How can I make Plank Pose more challenging?

To make Plank Pose more challenging, perform the pose as described in the steps below and then inhale as you lift one leg parallel to the floor. Remember to lengthen your body from the crown of your head and out through the sole of your raised foot. Hold your leg in this position for 10 to 20 seconds and then exhale as you lower your foot to the floor. Repeat this variation with your other leg raised.

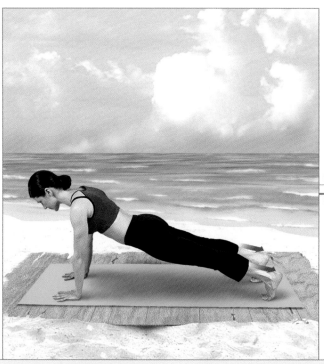

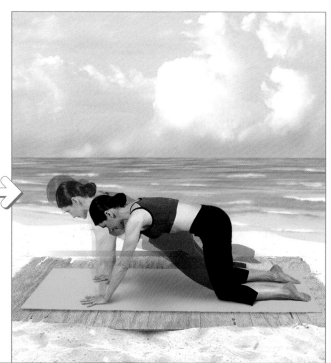

5 Extend your heels away from your body.

6 Move your shoulders down and back.

• You should keep your body straight. Do not allow your chest or pelvis to drop down or your buttocks to rise up.

• Make sure you keep your head in line with your spine.

• Visualize your body lengthening from the crown of your head to the soles of your feet.

7 Hold the pose for 10 to 20 seconds.

8 To come out of the pose, exhale as you bend your knees and return to Table Pose.

• After performing Plank Pose, you should perform a forward bend, such as Child's Pose, to release your spine and rest your arms.

eight point pose *(ashtanga namaskar)*

Eight Point Pose provides a good stretch for the front of your neck and your upper back. This pose also strengthens your chest, upper back, shoulders and arms.

As the name of the pose implies, eight parts of your body should be touching the floor as you hold the pose: your chin, your chest, two hands, two knees and two feet. It is important that your abdomen does not touch the floor while holding the pose. With these parts of your body touching the floor, this pose

provides a gentle upper back bend that is not found in many other poses.

Eight Point Pose serves as a great transition from Table Pose to Upward-Facing Dog Pose or Cobra Pose, and is commonly performed as part of Sun Salutation.

If you feel pressure on your knees in this pose, you can place a folded towel or blanket under your knees.

Use caution performing this pose if you have neck, shoulder, back, elbow or wrist problems.

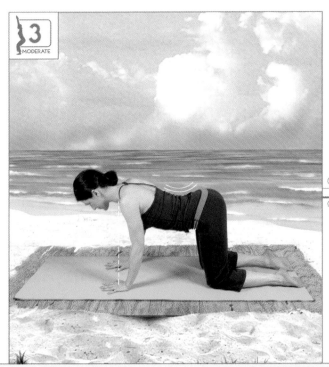

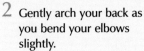

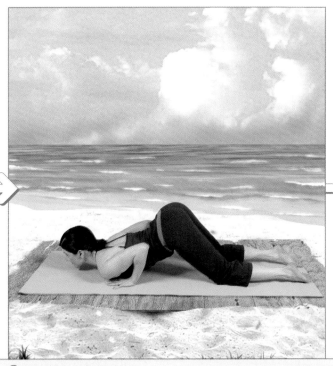

1 Begin in Table Pose. For information on Table Pose, see page 172.

- Make sure your hands are directly below your shoulders.

2 Gently arch your back as you bend your elbows slightly.

3 Exhale as you lower your chest to the floor between your hands.

- You may need to adjust the position of your knees to allow your chest to rest on the floor.

CHAPTER 10: Table Poses

I have difficulty holding this pose. What can I do?

If your upper body is not strong enough to hold this pose, rest your forearms on the floor.

What can I do if my neck and throat feel strained in this pose?

You can try placing your forehead on the floor instead of placing your chin on the floor. Although this modification helps to reduce strain on your neck and throat, some beginners may find resting their forehead on the floor difficult.

How can I use this pose to build even more upper body strength?

To further strengthen your upper body in this pose, you can move back and forth between Table Pose and Eight Point Pose several times. Make sure you exhale as you move into Eight Point Pose and inhale as you move back into Table Pose.

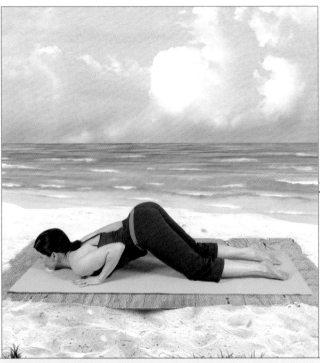

4 Stretch the front of your neck and place your chin on the floor.

• Your face should be looking forward.

5 Move your shoulder blades down and back.

• Make sure your elbows are close to your sides.

6 Curl your toes under and place the balls of your feet on the floor.

7 Press your tailbone toward the ceiling to lengthen your spine.

8 Hold the pose for 15 to 30 seconds.

• After performing Eight Point Pose, you should perform a counter pose, such as Crocodile Pose, to rest your spine.

downward-facing
dog pose *(adho mukha svanasana)*

Downward-Facing Dog Pose lengthens your spine and provides an intense stretch to the back of your legs, with an emphasis on stretching your calves. You can perform Downward-Facing Dog Pose to warm up your legs in preparation for other poses.

While performing Downward-Facing Dog Pose, focus on shifting your weight back onto your legs. Resting most of your weight on your legs helps to relieve the pressure on your arms, which is especially useful if you have shoulder or wrist problems. As you shift

your weight back, concentrate on stretching your heels toward the floor. If the back of your legs are tight, do not expect your heels to touch the floor.

As you perform the pose, keep your shoulder blades wide and your spine lengthened. You should also try to establish one straight line with your arms and spine and another with your legs, but make sure you do not lock your elbows or knees. To form these straight lines, try visualizing your body making an upside down V shape.

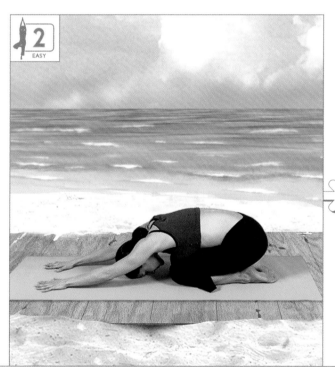

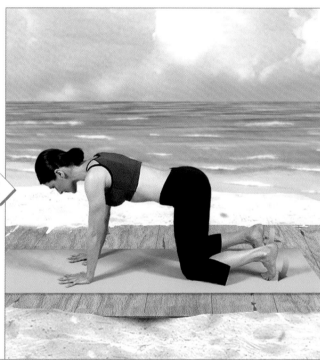

1 Begin in Child's Pose. For information on Child's Pose, see page 106.

2 Stretch your arms straight out in front of you, with your hands shoulder width apart.

3 Spread your fingers out and press your palms into the floor.

4 While maintaining the position of your hands, come up onto your hands and knees into Table Pose. For more information on Table Pose, see page 172. Your knees should be hip width apart.

5 Tuck your toes under.

The back of my legs feel strained. Should I continue performing the pose?

If the back of your legs feel strained in Downward-Facing Dog Pose, you can continue the pose, but bend your knees slightly. Even with this modification, you can still feel a deep stretch along the back of your legs. You can try straightening your legs a little more each time you perform the pose.

How can I modify the pose if I have wrist problems?

If you have wrist problems, you can try placing your knuckles, instead of your palms, on the floor as you perform Downward-Facing Dog Pose. You can also try performing the pose with your wrists supported. To support your wrists, place a rolled up towel under your wrists and allow your fingers to rest on the floor.

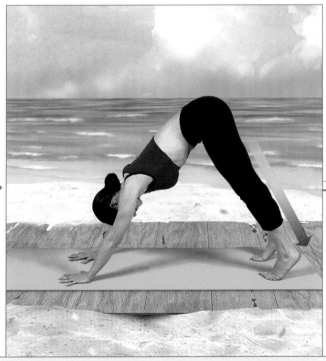

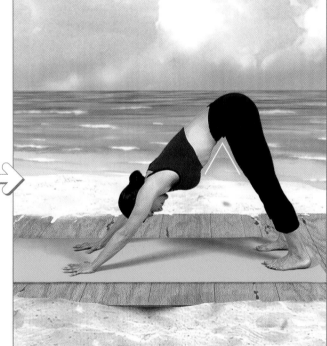

6 Exhale as you lift your hips and straighten your legs.

7 Exhale as you shift your weight back onto your legs and stretch your heels toward the floor.

8 Relax your head and neck toward the floor as your spine lengthens.

• Visualize your body making an upside down V shape.

9 Hold the pose for 1 to 3 minutes.

• To come out of the pose, exhale as you bend your knees to the floor and then return to Child's Pose.

Chapter 11

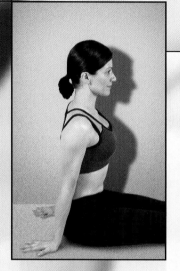

Back bends can be intense and challenging, but they are useful for strengthening and aligning your spine. Back bends are also beneficial because they open the front of your body, particularly your chest, which can help improve your breathing. This chapter demonstrates back bends you can perform to keep your spine strong and supple. Make sure you always perform a forward bend after a back bend to release your lower back and return your spine to a neutral position.

Back Bends

In this Chapter...

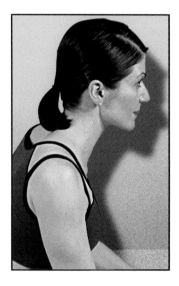

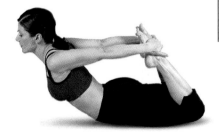

standing back bend

You can perform Standing Back Bend to open and stretch the front of your body. This pose also strengthens your abdominal muscles and back, with an emphasis on your lower back. You can perform Standing Back Bend to help you learn correct spinal alignment, which can alleviate problems with your spine.

Standing Back Bend is a good warm-up pose for other standing poses, such as Dancer Pose. This pose is also commonly performed as part of Sun Salutation.

As you hold the pose, do not allow your head to drop back or your lower back to arch too much. Instead, try to maintain length through your entire spine as you visualize the smooth and gentle curve of your back.

After performing Standing Back Bend, you should perform a standing forward bend, such as Rag Doll Pose, to stretch your spine in the opposite direction.

You should use caution performing Standing Back Bend if you have problems with your neck or lower back.

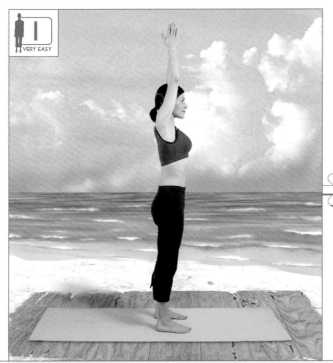

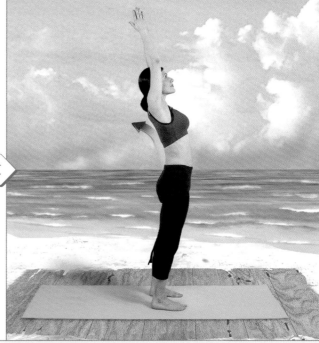

VERY EASY

1 Begin in Mountain Pose. For information on Mountain Pose, see page 120.

2 Inhale as you circle your arms out to each side and bring your palms together overhead.

• Your arms should be straight, but your elbows should not be locked.

3 Relax your shoulders down away from your ears.

4 Press your feet into the floor and extend through the crown of your head to lengthen your spine.

5 Inhale as you press your hips forward and gently arch your upper body backward.

• Make sure you keep your head and neck in line with your spine.

• Your upper arms should stay beside your ears throughout the pose.

My lower back feels strained in this pose. What can I do?

To make this pose easier on your lower back, you can stand with your legs a little wider than hip width apart. You can also try standing straight with your arms extended overhead, instead of bending backward. While standing straight, focus on lengthening your entire body and move your upper arms back slightly behind your ears to open the front of your body.

How can I open my chest more in this pose?

To open your chest more, step your right foot forward and clasp your elbows behind your back. Then inhale as you gently arch your upper back backwards. After holding the pose for 15 to 45 seconds, inhale as you lift your torso upright and then exhale as you return to Mountain Pose. Repeat these steps with your left foot forward. If you cannot lie on your stomach, this variation serves as a good alternative to Cobra Pose.

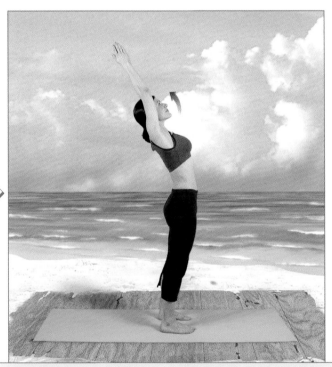

MODIFICATION

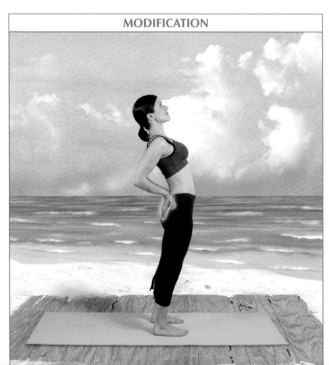

6 Tilt your head to look up at the ceiling, keeping your neck long.

• Make sure you do not allow your head to drop back.

7 Hold the pose for 5 to 30 seconds.

8 To come out of the pose, inhale and lift your torso upright. Then exhale and bring your arms to your sides.

• You can perform Standing Back Bend with your hands on your lower back to help support your lower back. This modification also allows you to support some of your weight with your arms.

1 Perform Standing Back Bend, except place your palms on your lower back with your fingers pointing toward the floor.

sphinx pose

Sphinx Pose is a basic back bend that helps to develop strength and flexibility in your spine and back, with an emphasis on your lower back. You can use this pose to open your chest to help increase your lung capacity. This pose is also useful for stimulating your nervous system to energize your body.

As you perform this pose, try to focus on the way your body feels. Developing an awareness of your body in Sphinx Pose can help you learn how to perform other back bends correctly. This pose can also help you build the strength and flexibility in your back and spine that you need to perform more difficult back bends, such as Cobra Pose.

While performing Sphinx Pose, make sure your elbows are directly under your shoulders. You should also focus on lifting through your chest as your forearms support your upper body.

Avoid performing Sphinx Pose if you have back, arm or shoulder problems.

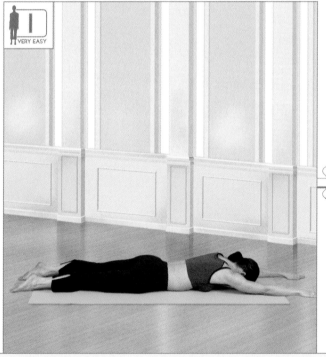

VERY EASY

1 Lie face down with your legs extended behind you and your feet hip width apart. Rest the top of your feet on the floor.

2 Stretch your arms straight in front of you, with your palms facing down.

3 Rest your forehead on the floor.

4 Bend your elbows and slide your hands back toward you.

• Your elbows should be directly under your shoulders and your forearms should be flat on the floor.

5 Spread your fingers out, with your middle fingers pointing straight ahead.

6 Lift your chest forward. Feel your chest opening and expanding with each breath.

What should I do if my lower back feels strained in Sphinx Pose?

To reduce the strain in your lower back, place a folded blanket under your abdomen, just above your pubic bone. As you perform the pose, your pubic bone should still be able to rest on the floor. This modification also helps you lift your upper body into the pose.

How can I stretch my neck in Sphinx Pose?

As you hold the pose, you can perform a neck stretch. Keeping the crown of your head pointing toward the ceiling, turn your head to the right and look over your right shoulder for 5 to 10 seconds. Then turn your head to the left and look over your left shoulder for another 5 to 10 seconds.

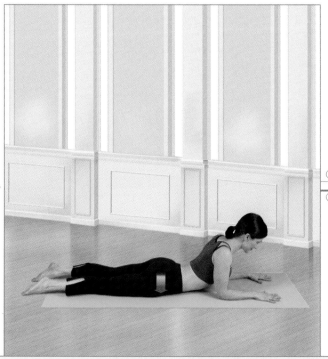

7 Exhale as you gently press your hips and pelvis into the floor.

- Make sure you keep your hips and pelvis pressed to the floor throughout the pose, but do not squeeze your buttocks.

- Make sure you maintain length through your neck and keep your shoulders back and down as you lengthen your spine.

8 Point the crown of your head toward the ceiling and gaze straight ahead.

- Visualize the long, even curve of your spine as you rest, like the Sphinx, in the desert sand.

9 Hold the pose for 15 seconds to 1 minute.

- After performing Sphinx Pose, you should perform a forward bend, such as Child's Pose, to release your lower back.

cobra pose *(bhujangasana)*

Cobra Pose develops strength and flexibility in your spine and back, with an emphasis on your lower back.

While performing daily tasks, most people bend forward more often than they bend backward. Cobra Pose acts as a counterbalance to this tendency to bend forward, helping to keep your spine strong and supple. This pose also opens your chest to help increase your lung capacity and stimulates your nervous system to invigorate your body.

Your lower back is vulnerable to compression because

it is the easiest part of your spine to bend. To avoid compressing your lower back, make sure you lengthen through your entire spine as you curl your spine up.

Although your arms support your upper body in this pose, you should only lift your upper body using your spine, not your arms. Continue to straighten your arms only while you feel your spine lengthening and you can keep your shoulders and elbows relaxed.

Avoid performing Cobra Pose if you have back problems.

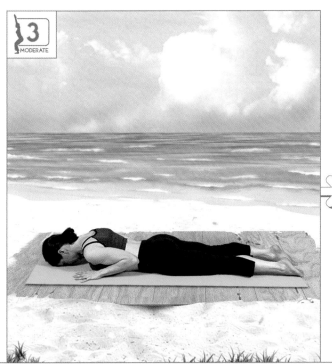

3 MODERATE

1 Lie flat on the floor with your legs no wider than hip width apart. Your forehead and the top of your feet should be resting on the floor.

2 Place your palms on the floor under your shoulders.

3 Spread your fingers out, with your middle fingers pointing straight ahead.

- Your elbows should be close to your sides.

4 Exhale as you gently press your pelvis toward the floor.

- Make sure you keep your pelvis pressed into the floor throughout the pose, but do not squeeze your buttocks.

5 Inhale as you begin to curl your spine up, one vertebra at a time.

6 Slowly lift your forehead, nose and chin off the floor. Then raise your head to look forward.

My spine is stiff. Can I still perform Cobra Pose?

If your spine is stiff, you may want to perform an easier back bend, such as Sphinx Pose, to build up strength and flexibility in your spine. For information on Sphinx Pose, see page 194. When you are ready to try Cobra Pose, you should perform a modified version of the pose. When going into Cobra Pose, place your palms on the floor in front of your shoulders, instead of under your shoulders. This modification lengthens your spine, which helps ensure you do not strain your back.

Can I modify Cobra Pose to incorporate movement?

Yes. As you perform Cobra Pose, you can move your upper body up and down with your breath. Inhale as you slowly lift your chest off the floor and then exhale as you slowly lower your chest back down to the floor. You can repeat this movement three to five times and then hold the pose. Incorporating movement into Cobra Pose can help you further elongate your spine before holding the pose.

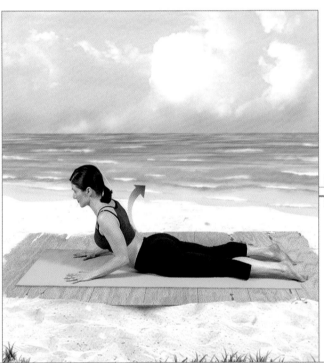

7 Continue curling your spine up to bring your chest off the floor.

- Make sure you maintain length through your neck and keep your shoulders back and down as you curl your spine.

8 Press your hands into the floor and slowly straighten your arms to help lift your upper body further off the floor.

- Make sure you do not use the strength of your arms to lift your upper body.

9 Point the crown of your head toward the ceiling and gaze straight ahead.

- Visualize the long, even curve of your spine.

10 Hold the pose for 5 to 15 seconds.

- After performing Cobra Pose, you should perform a forward bend, such as Child's Pose, to release your lower back.

upward-facing
dog pose *(urdhva mukha svanasana)*

Upward-Facing Dog Pose is a back bend that opens your chest and helps to strengthen your upper body. This pose also provides an intense stretch for your shoulders, arms, wrists, abdomen and lower back.

Upward-Facing Dog Pose is often performed as part of Sun Salutation. For information on Sun Salutation, see page 262.

As you straighten your arms to lift your upper body away from the floor in this pose, make sure your spine is lengthened to avoid compressing your lower back.

You should also allow your neck to follow the curve of your spine and make sure your shoulders are relaxed down. It is more important to relax and widen your shoulders than it is to straighten your arms completely. Keeping your chest lifted and expanded as you hold Upward-Facing Dog Pose will also help you achieve the full benefits of the pose.

While performing this pose, try to visualize your chest opening and your body lengthening from the crown of your head to the tips of your toes.

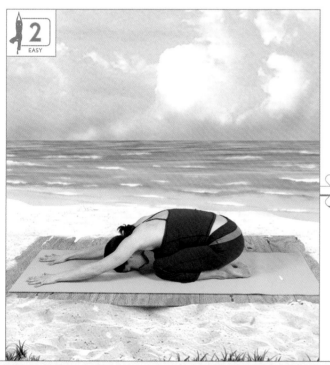 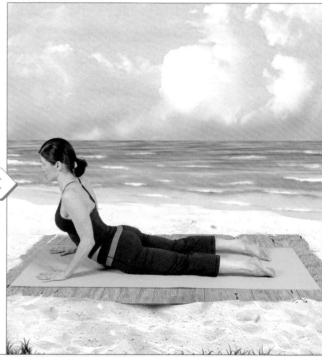

1 Begin in Child's Pose. For information on Child's Pose, see page 106.

2 Stretch your arms straight out in front of you, with your hands shoulder width apart.

3 Spread your fingers out, with your middle fingers pointing straight ahead.

4 Maintaining the position of your hands and knees, inhale as you press your palms into the floor and stretch your body forward along the floor.

5 Straighten your arms to lift your upper body and head away from the floor, keeping your neck relaxed.

• Make sure your hands are directly under your shoulders and your elbows are not locked.

When should I avoid performing this pose?

You should avoid performing Upward-Facing Dog Pose if you have wrist problems, such as Carpal Tunnel Syndrome, or lower back problems.

How can I deepen Upward-Facing Dog Pose?

You can tilt your head back slightly to look up at the ceiling as you hold the pose. Make sure you do not bend your neck too far backwards. Your neck should feel long and uncompressed. If you have a stiff or sore neck, do not perform this modification.

How can I make this pose easier?

To make Upward-Facing Dog Pose easier, perform the pose as described in the steps below, except leave the top of your feet and your lower legs on the floor. This modification is useful if you find the pose too intense, if your upper body is weak or injured or if you have problems with your feet or toes. You can practice this modification to help gain the upper body strength necessary to perform the pose with your toes tucked under.

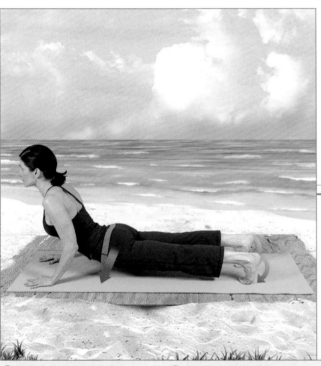
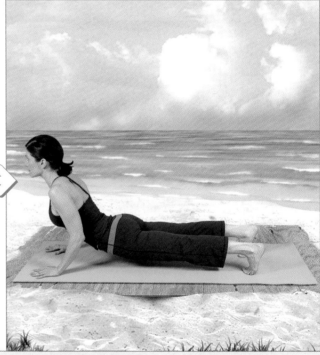

6 Press the front of your pelvis and your hips toward the floor.

7 Press down through your palms and then curl your toes under to place the balls of your feet on the floor.

8 Press down through the balls of your feet to lift your knees and lower legs off the floor.

9 Point the crown of your head toward the ceiling to lengthen your spine.

• Visualize your entire spine lengthening. Your lower back should not feel compressed.

10 Lift and expand your chest as you relax your shoulders down away from your ears.

11 Hold the pose for 5 to 30 seconds.

• To come out of the pose, exhale as you lower your legs to the floor and then return to Child's Pose.

front lying boat pose *(supta navasana)*

Front Lying Boat Pose strengthens your back, with an emphasis on strengthening your lower back. This pose also helps to develop your stamina and concentration.

As you lift your upper body and legs off the floor in this pose, make sure you keep your upper arms beside your ears and your hips on the floor. It is more important to create length through your arms and legs than to lift them higher up off the floor. Focus on stretching your fingers away from your shoulders and your toes away from your hips as you visualize your whole body lengthening.

You can modify this pose by lifting only one arm and one leg, which can be a useful warm-up exercise for the full pose. This modification helps to improve your coordination and teaches the two sides of your body to work independently.

Take care not to compress your lower back or strain your neck or shoulders in this pose. You should also be careful performing this pose if you have abdominal, back or neck problems.

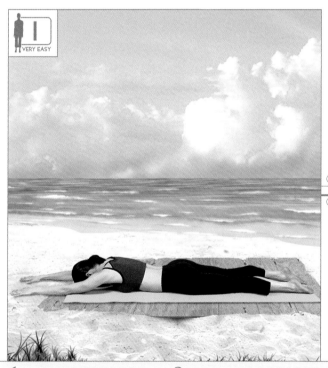

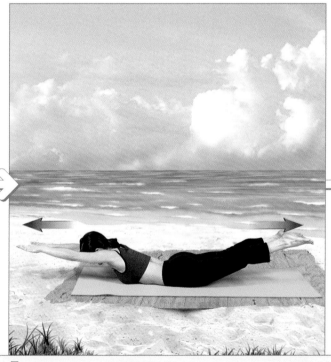

1 Lie face down with your legs extended behind you and your feet hip width apart. Rest the top of your feet on the floor.

2 Stretch your arms straight in front of you, with your palms facing down.

3 Rest your forehead on the floor.

4 Exhale as you press your hips and pelvis into the floor and then stretch both legs behind you.

5 Inhale as you lift your arms, chest, head and both legs up.

6 Reach out through your fingers, toes and the crown of your head. Keep your head in line with your spine.

- Lengthen through your torso, arms and legs.
- Make sure both hips remain on the floor and your legs are straight, but your knees are not locked.

How can I open my chest in this pose?

Interlace your fingers behind your back and then press your shoulder blades together. Then lift your arms up as you lift your chest, head and legs off the floor.

How can I build strength in my back so I can hold the pose longer?

You can come in and out of the pose a few times before you hold the pose to strengthen your back so you can hold the pose longer.

My shoulders feel strained in this pose. What can I do?

You can place your arms alongside your body, with your palms facing the floor. As you raise your chest and legs, lift your arms so they are parallel to the floor and look straight ahead.

You can also lift your arms to shoulder height and out to your sides, like the wings of an airplane, as you raise your chest and legs. This modification also helps to open your chest.

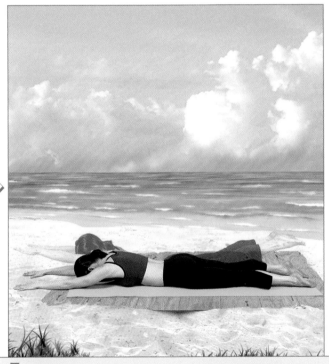

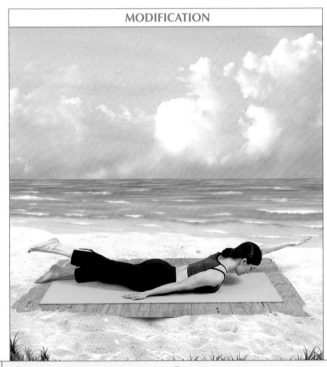

MODIFICATION

7 Hold the pose for 5 to 30 seconds.

8 To come out of the pose, exhale as you lower your upper body and legs to the floor. Then turn your head to one side and rest your cheek on the floor.

- After performing Front Lying Boat Pose, you should perform a forward bend, such as Child's Pose, to release your lower back.

1 You can perform Front Lying Boat Pose with only one arm and leg raised. Begin the pose with your right arm at your side and your left arm extended in front of you, both palms facing down.

2 Inhale as you raise your left arm, chest, head and right leg off the floor. Then exhale as you lower your arm, chest, head and leg.

3 Repeat the modification for your other arm and leg.

half locust pose *(ardha salabhasana)*

Half Locust Pose is beneficial for strengthening your legs and back, with an emphasis on strengthening your lower back. This pose also stimulates your abdominal organs, which can help improve digestion. You can use this pose to warm up for Locust Pose, which is a more advanced version of Half Locust Pose. For information on Locust Pose, see page 204.

While performing Half Locust Pose, you may find you can only lift your legs a few inches off the floor.

However, it is more important to create length through your legs than to try to lift your legs higher up off the floor. You may find it helpful to visualize your body lengthening through your spine and legs.

Make sure you do not strain your neck and shoulders while performing Half Locust Pose. You should also avoid compressing your lower back in this pose. Do not perform this pose if you have a back or neck injury.

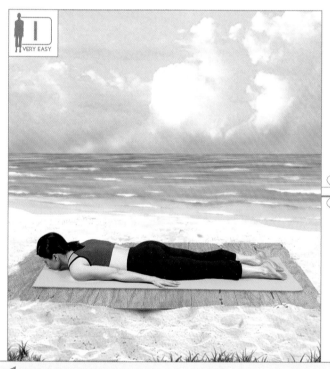

VERY EASY

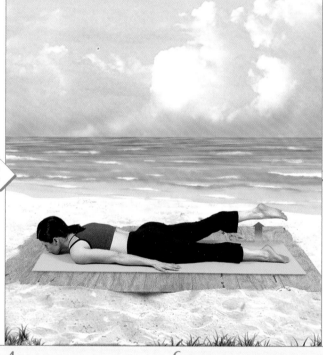

1 Lie face down with your legs extended behind you. Rest the top of your feet on the floor hip width apart.

2 Place your arms alongside your body, palms down. Extend your fingers toward your feet to lengthen your arms.

• Make sure your arms are straight and your shoulders are relaxed down away from your ears.

3 Rest your chin on the floor.

4 Exhale as you press your hips and pelvis into the floor.

5 Stretch your right leg behind you.

6 Inhale as you lift your right leg up toward the ceiling.

• Make sure you keep your chin on the floor as you lift your leg.

What can I do if I have trouble lifting my legs in this pose?

Place a folded blanket under your pelvis to reduce the stress on your lower back. You should have an easier time lifting your legs when your pelvis is supported.

I feel pressure on the front of my body in this pose. What can I do?

You can lay your body on a folded blanket to provide a cushion between your body and the floor.

What should I do if my neck feels strained?

If your neck feels strained, you can place your forehead on the floor instead of your chin. You can also turn your head to rest your cheek on the floor. Make sure you turn your head away from the leg you are lifting. For example, if you are lifting your right leg, turn your head to the left and rest your right cheek on the floor. If you find resting your cheek on the floor uncomfortable, fold your arms in front of you and rest your cheek on your arms.

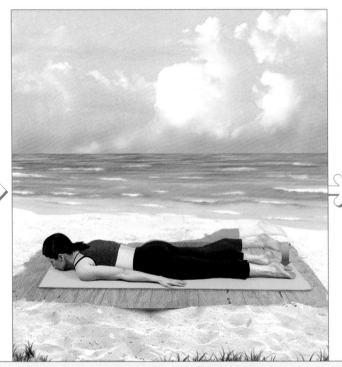

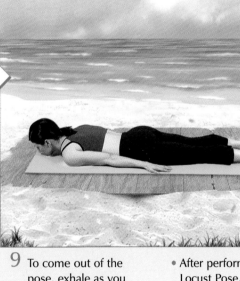

- Make sure you keep both hips on the floor. Your legs should be straight, but your knees should not be locked.

- Visualize your spine lengthening and your foot and toes moving away from your hip.

7 Exhale as you lower your leg to the floor.

8 Lift and lower your leg three times and then hold the pose with your leg raised for 5 to 15 seconds.

9 To come out of the pose, exhale as you lower your leg to the floor.

10 Repeat steps 4 to 9 for your other side.

- After performing Half Locust Pose, you should perform a forward bend, such as Child's Pose, to release your lower back.

locust pose *(salabhasana)*

Locust Pose is beneficial for strengthening your legs and back, with an emphasis on strengthening your lower back. This pose also stimulates your abdominal organs, which can help improve digestion.

Do not be concerned if you can only lift your legs a few inches off the floor in this pose. It is more important to create length through your legs than to try to lift your legs higher up off the floor. You should try to visualize your body lengthening through your spine and legs as you stretch your toes away from your

hips. As you lift your legs in this pose, make sure you do not compress your lower back or strain your neck and shoulders.

If you experience discomfort in your neck, you can practice Half Locust Pose to help build the strength and flexibility required for Locust Pose. For information on Half Locust Pose, see page 202.

Do not perform this pose if you have a back or neck injury or if you have abdominal problems.

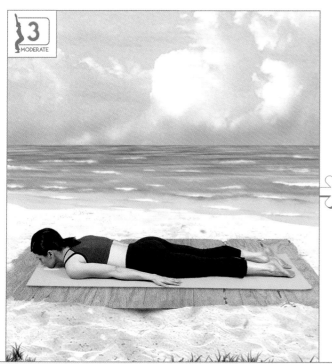

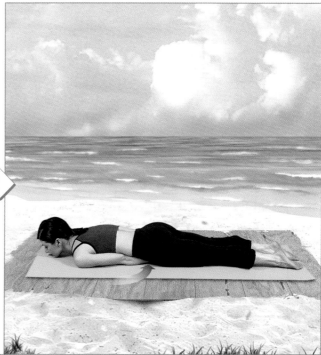

1 Lie face down with your legs extended behind you. Rest the top of your feet on the floor no wider than hip width apart.

2 Place your arms on the floor alongside your body, with your palms facing the floor.

3 Rest your chin on the floor.

4 Rock your body from side to side to walk your arms under your body. Then interlace your fingers.

• Your forearms should be inside your hip bones and your elbows should be as close together as possible.

5 Relax your shoulders and extend your hands toward your feet to lengthen your arms.

6 Exhale as you press your hips and pelvis toward the floor.

Do I have to tuck my arms under my body in this pose?

No. If you do not have a lot of flexibility in your arms and shoulders, you can leave your arms alongside your body with your palms facing the floor. This modification is also useful if you find tucking your arms under your body uncomfortable.

What can I do if I have trouble lifting my legs in this pose?

You can place a folded blanket under your pelvis to reduce the stress on your lower back. You should find lifting your legs easier when your pelvis is supported.

How can I reduce the pressure on my pelvis and hands in this pose?

Perform the pose as described below, except make your hands into fists and rest the back of your hands on the floor under your thighs.

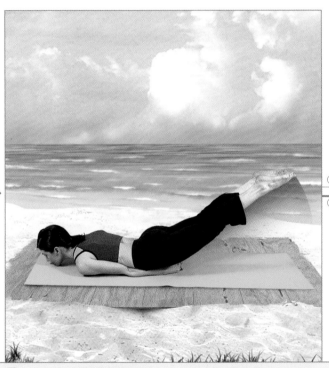

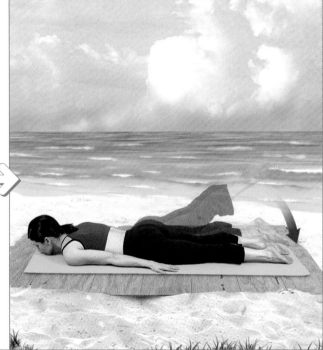

7 Stretch both legs behind you and then inhale as you lift both legs up toward the ceiling.

- Keep your legs straight, but do not lock your knees. Your feet should be hip width apart.

- Your hips, knees and the top of your feet should be facing down.

- Make sure you keep your chin on the floor.

8 Press your arms and hands into the floor.

9 Hold the pose for 5 to 30 seconds.

10 To come out of the pose, exhale as you lower your legs to the floor. Then turn your head to one side and slide your arms out from under your body.

- After performing Locust Pose, you should perform a forward bend, such as Child's Pose, to release your lower back.

bow pose *(dhanurasana)*

Bow Pose is an advanced back bend that increases the strength and flexibility of your back and spine. In addition, Bow Pose stretches your abdominals, hips and the front of your shoulders and thighs. This invigorating pose also opens your chest, which can help improve your breathing.

Since this pose is an advanced back bend, you should gain experience with easier back bends, such as Bridge Pose, before you attempt Bow Pose. For information on Bridge Pose, see page 208.

In Bow Pose, stretching your legs away from your body helps to lift your head, chest and thighs off the floor. As your upper body lifts off the floor, keep your shoulders broad as you concentrate on lengthening your spine and using your entire spine to bend backward. If your lower back feels compressed, release your body down a bit or come out of the pose.

Always take caution when performing Bow Pose. You should avoid Bow Pose if you have back problems or high blood pressure.

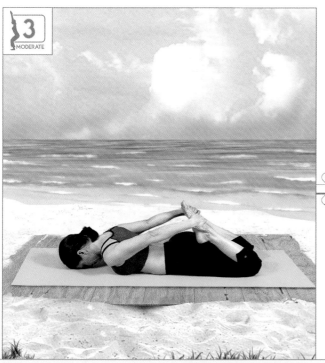
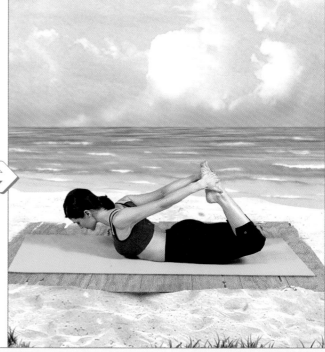

1 Lie flat on the floor with your forehead resting on the floor.

2 Bend your knees as you reach back with your hands and clasp your ankles or the top of your feet. Your knees and feet should be hip width apart.

3 Exhale as you gently press your pubic bone into the floor.

4 Inhale as you lift your head, chest and thighs off the floor.

5 Stretch your legs away from your body and press your feet into your hands to further lift your head, chest and thighs off the floor.

• Make sure your arms are straight, but your elbows are not locked.

I cannot clasp my ankles or feet in Bow Pose. What can I do?

You can loop a strap around the top of each foot and then grasp the ends of each strap in either hand. Keep the straps taut, but do not use the straps to pull yourself into the back bend. If you only have one strap, you can loop the strap around both of your feet. Remember to keep your knees and feet hip width apart when using straps.

How can I gain the flexibility needed to perform Bow Pose?

In addition to practicing easier back bends, you can perform Bow Pose holding only one leg at a time. Perform the pose as described in the steps below, except bend one knee and clasp your ankle or the top of your foot, as you keep your other leg straight and flat on the floor. Hold the pose for 10 to 30 seconds and then repeat the modification holding your other leg. Once you have gained more flexibility, you can try performing Bow Pose holding both legs.

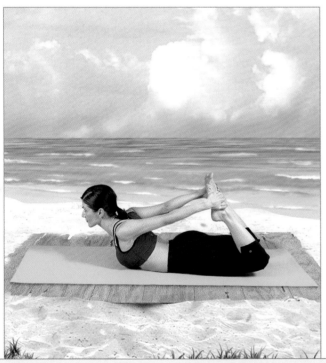

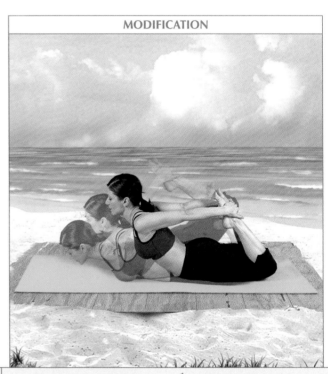

MODIFICATION

6 Point the crown of your head toward the ceiling and gaze straight ahead.

- Visualize your body forming a graceful bow with your arms as the string.

7 Hold the pose for 10 to 30 seconds and then exhale as you come out of the pose.

- After performing Bow Pose, you should perform a forward bend, such as Child's Pose, to release your lower back.

- You can modify Bow Pose to add movement to the pose and massage your abdominal organs.

1 Perform Bow Pose and then rock your body forward and backward three to five times before holding the pose. This modification is known as Rocking Bow.

bridge pose *(setu bhandasana)*

Bridge Pose is a basic back bend that opens your chest and strengthens your back. This pose also increases the flexibility of your spine and stretches your neck, abdomen and thighs. As with all back bends, this pose can help energize your body, which makes the pose a good warm-up pose.

While performing Bridge Pose, make sure your weight is resting equally on your shoulders and feet. You should also relax your shoulders away from your ears, but be careful not to overstretch your neck. As you

hold the pose, focus on breathing and lengthening your spine as you arch your body like a bridge.

If you want to deepen the pose, you can move your shoulder blades toward each other. Then interlace your fingers and gently stretch your arms and hands toward your feet.

You should be careful performing Bridge Pose if you have neck, shoulder, back or knee problems. Avoid the pose completely if you have a serious knee injury, high blood pressure or heart disease.

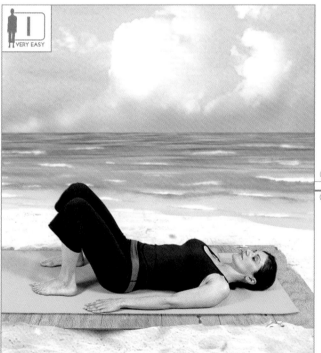

VERY EASY

1 Lie on your back with your knees bent and your feet flat on the floor, hip width apart with your heels directly under your knees.

• Make sure your knees and toes are pointing forward.

2 Place your arms on the floor along the sides of your body, with your palms facing down.

3 Exhale as you lengthen your spine and gently press your lower back into the floor.

4 Inhale as you press your feet into the floor and lift your pelvis off the floor as high as is comfortable for you.

• Your weight should be supported equally by your shoulders and feet.

• If you feel any discomfort in your neck or shoulders, you should come out of the pose.

I find it difficult to keep my pelvis lifted in Bridge Pose. What can I do?

If you find it difficult to keep your pelvis lifted in this pose, you can position a prop, such as a bolster, under your lower back and rest the back of your pelvis on the prop. This modification is especially helpful if you cannot lift your pelvis up very high in this pose. Resting the back of your pelvis on a prop will also allow you to hold the pose for a longer period of time.

Is there anything else I can do to hold Bridge Pose longer?

To stay in Bridge Pose longer, you can use your hands to support your pelvis. Instead of placing your arms along the sides of your body, bend your elbows and place your hands on your lower back, keeping your upper arms on the floor. You may only be able to perform this modification if you are very flexible. If you have wrist or arm problems, you should avoid this modification.

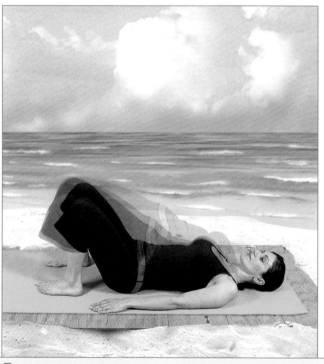

MODIFICATION

5 Hold the pose for 30 seconds to 1 minute.

6 To come out of the pose, exhale as you roll your spine down to the floor one vertebra at a time. Your hips should touch the floor last.

• After performing Bridge Pose, you should perform Little Boat Pose to release your lower back. For information on Little Boat Pose, see page 58.

• You can intensify the stretch in your chest and add a gentle stretch to your arms and shoulders in Bridge Pose.

1 Perform Bridge Pose, except move your shoulder blades toward each other. Keeping your arms on the floor, interlace your fingers and gently stretch your arms and hands toward your feet.

fish pose *(matsyasana)*

Fish Pose is a calming pose that provides a good stretch for your neck and upper back. You can also use this pose to increase the flexibility of your spine and release tension in your back. This pose is also beneficial for opening your chest to facilitate deep breathing, which is especially useful for asthmatics.

You may want to perform Fish Pose as a counter pose for Shoulderstand or Plow Pose because the pose stretches your neck in the opposite direction.

While performing Fish Pose, make sure your elbows support the weight of your body, while the crown of your head rests lightly on the floor. You should never feel any pressure on your head or strain in your neck. As you hold the pose, focus on keeping the curve of your spine smooth and even from the crown of your head to your tailbone.

You should use caution performing this pose if you have problems with your neck, shoulders, arms or back.

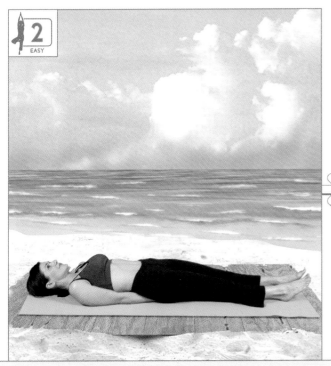

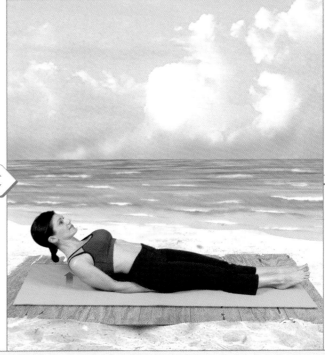

1 Begin in Relaxation Pose. For information on Relaxation Pose, see page 242.

2 Bring your feet and legs together.

3 Rock your body from side to side to tuck your arms under your body and position your palms face down underneath you.

• Your arms should be straight, but your elbows should not be locked.

4 Inhale and press your elbows into the floor to raise your upper body off the floor.

• Make sure you keep your neck and shoulders relaxed. Your spine, neck and head should be in a straight line.

• Your legs should be straight, but your knees should not be locked.

What can I do if I have difficulty lifting my upper body into the pose?

Place a prop, such as a bolster or rolled blanket, under your shoulder blades. Lower the crown of your head to the floor and extend your arms out to the sides at shoulder height with your palms facing up. You may also need to position another prop under your neck to support your neck and head. Your head should follow the curve of your spine and you should not feel any strain in your neck.

Is there an easier alternative to Fish Pose that provides similar benefits?

Yes. Begin in Staff Pose, as shown on page 72, with your palms on the floor behind your hips and your fingers pointing behind you. Lift and round your chest and look toward the ceiling, keeping your neck elongated.

How can I stretch my inner thighs and hips in Fish Pose?

Begin in Easy Pose, as shown on page 74, and then lower your upper body to the floor to perform the pose.

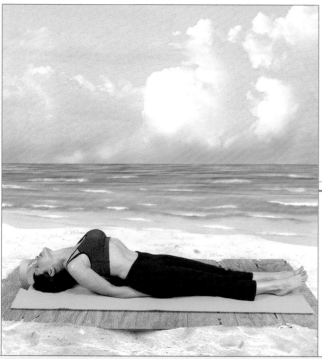

5 Exhale and lower the crown of your head to the floor.

• Make sure your weight is supported by your elbows. The top of your head should rest lightly on the floor.

• Visualize the strong arch in your upper back and the width of your chest expanding.

6 Hold the pose for 15 seconds to 1 minute.

7 To come out of the pose, press your elbows into the floor and lift your head. Then lower your back to the floor one vertebra at a time.

8 After performing Fish Pose, you should gently roll your head from side to side to relax your neck muscles.

inclined
plane pose *(purvottanasana)*

Inclined Plane Pose is an energizing pose that strengthens your entire body, with an emphasis on strengthening your upper body. This pose provides a good stretch to the front of your body, which helps to open your chest and improve the flexibility of your shoulders. You can also use this pose to relieve tension in your neck and shoulders.

If you find it difficult to place your palms shoulder width apart in this pose, you can place your palms as

close together as is comfortable for you. Once your palms are in a comfortable position, make sure your body forms a straight line from your shoulders down to your feet. Do not allow your buttocks to drop toward the floor.

Use caution performing this pose if you have an injury to your neck, arms or shoulders. Also, be careful performing this pose if you have a wrist injury, such as Carpal Tunnel Syndrome.

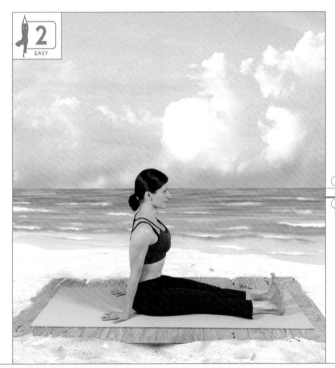

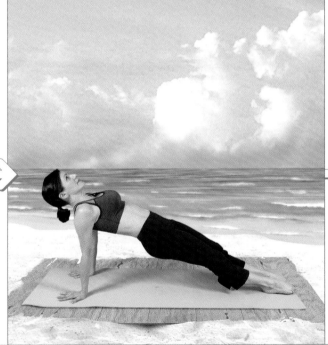

1 Begin in Staff Pose. For information on Staff Pose, see page 72.

2 Place your palms on the floor behind your hips, shoulder width apart.

• Your fingers should be pointing away from you.

3 Press your palms and heels into the floor.

4 Inhale as you lift your hips toward the ceiling.

• Your wrists should be directly below your shoulders.

5 Press the soles of your feet toward the floor.

How can I reduce the weight on my arms and wrists in this pose?

Begin the pose with your knees bent, hip width apart and your feet flat on the floor. After you press your palms into the floor and lift your hips toward the ceiling, keep your knees bent to allow your feet to support some of your weight.

My neck feels strained in this pose. What can I do?

To reduce the strain on your neck, perform the pose with your chin tucked into your chest instead of dropping your head back.

What can I do if I find Inclined Plane Pose too difficult?

Perform steps 1 and 2 below and then inhale as you lift your chest and look up at the ceiling without dropping your head back. Make sure you keep your hips on the floor.

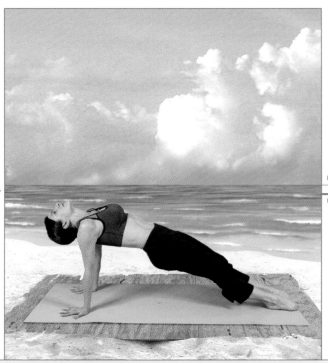

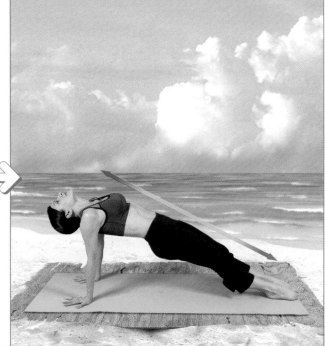

6 Relax your neck and allow your head to gently drop back.

- Keep your body straight. You should not allow your buttocks to drop down.

- Visualize your body lengthening from your shoulders to the soles of your feet.

7 Hold the pose for 5 to 20 seconds.

8 To come out of the pose, exhale as you lower your hips to the floor.

- After performing Inclined Plane Pose, you should shake out your hands to help relieve your wrists.

camel
pose (ustrasana)

Camel Pose is an advanced back bend that helps to open your chest and the front of your body. This pose also strengthens your back and spine, while providing an intense stretch to the front of your thighs.

As you stretch backward into the pose, try to keep your thighs perpendicular to the floor. Also, be careful not to drop your head back because this can compress the back of your neck. Your neck should stay in line with the curve of your spine. If you feel any strain in your neck, you can tuck your chin toward your chest as you hold the pose. When coming out of the pose, you should relax your neck and lift your upper body before you return your head to an upright position.

If kneeling on the floor is uncomfortable for you, you can place a blanket under your knees and feet. You should use caution when performing Camel Pose if you have a hernia or problems with your neck, shoulders, back or knees.

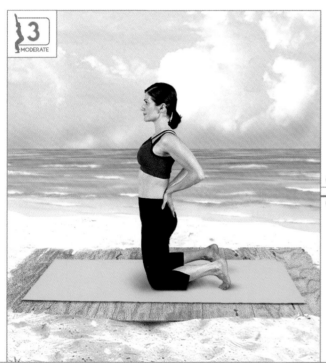

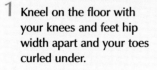

1 Kneel on the floor with your knees and feet hip width apart and your toes curled under.

2 Place your hands on your lower back, with your fingers pointing down.

3 Press your thighs and the front of your pelvis forward, while you tuck your tailbone down and under.

4 Inhale as you lift your ribcage and lengthen through your spine.

5 Press your shoulders back and allow your upper arms to follow.

6 Lift your heart toward the ceiling and then bend your upper body backward.

- You should try to bend from as high in your back as possible.

What can I do if I cannot reach my feet in this pose?

You can position blocks vertically on either side of your feet and rest your hands on the blocks.

How can I deepen Camel Pose?

Rest the top of your feet on the floor and point your toes behind you, instead of curling your toes under. You will need to stretch further down to reach your heels in this modification, so be careful not to compress your lower back.

How can I open my chest and the front of my body more in this pose?

Perform the pose as described in the steps below, except reach only one hand back to your foot and then stretch your other hand above your head so your upper arm is beside your ear. Make sure you keep your thighs as perpendicular to the floor as possible. Repeat this modification for your other side.

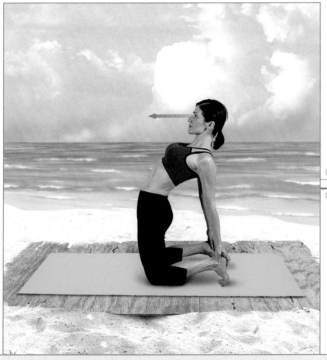

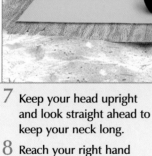

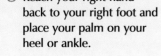

7 Keep your head upright and look straight ahead to keep your neck long.

8 Reach your right hand back to your right foot and place your palm on your heel or ankle.

9 Reach your left hand back to your left foot and place your palm on your heel or ankle.

• Try to keep your thighs as perpendicular to the floor as possible.

10 Lengthen the back of your neck and then tilt your head to look up at the ceiling. Make sure you keep your neck long.

11 Hold the pose for 30 seconds to 1 minute.

12 To come out of the pose, inhale as you lift your upper body and return to a kneeling position.

• After performing Camel Pose, you should perform a forward bend, such as Child's Pose, to release your spine.

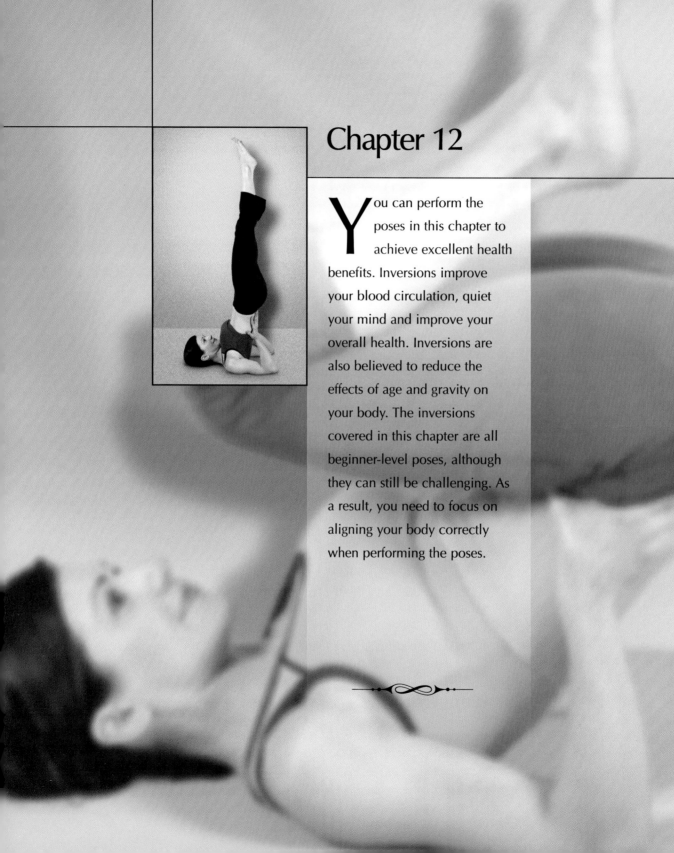

Chapter 12

Y ou can perform the poses in this chapter to achieve excellent health benefits. Inversions improve your blood circulation, quiet your mind and improve your overall health. Inversions are also believed to reduce the effects of age and gravity on your body. The inversions covered in this chapter are all beginner-level poses, although they can still be challenging. As a result, you need to focus on aligning your body correctly when performing the poses.

Inversions

In this Chapter...

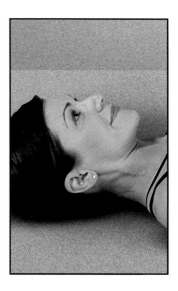

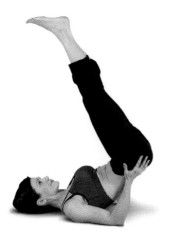

legs up the wall
pose *(viparita karani)*

Legs Up the Wall Pose is a restorative pose that helps reduce tension in your head, neck and shoulders and improves your circulation. This pose can also help reduce stress, lower your blood pressure, help relieve insomnia and relieve tiredness in your legs and feet.

It is important to correctly align your spine in Legs Up the Wall Pose. To ensure your spine is straight, keep your head in line with your spine and your shoulders in line with your hips.

If your legs feel tight in this pose, try sitting farther away from the wall. If you are more flexible, you can sit closer to the wall. Once you find the distance that is most comfortable for you, make sure your legs and upper body feel fully supported by the wall and floor.

Avoid this pose if you have neck or back problems, low blood pressure or if you are menstruating. Also, use caution performing this pose if you have eye problems, such as glaucoma.

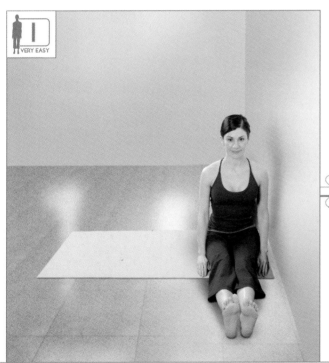

VERY EASY

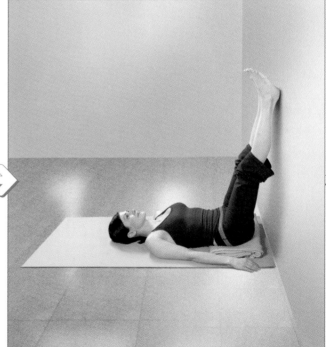

1 Position a folded blanket approximately 3 inches away from a wall.

2 Sit on the blanket beside the wall, with your legs extended and your left side facing the wall.

3 Lower your upper body to the floor as you swing your legs up onto the wall.

- Your hips should be comfortably resting on the blanket. Your shoulders should be resting on the floor.

- Make sure your legs are straight but your knees are not locked. Your feet should be hip width apart.

Can I stretch my inner thighs while performing Legs Up the Wall Pose?

Yes. You can modify the pose to provide a stretch to your inner thighs. Perform the pose as described below, except separate your legs until they form a V shape on the wall.

I adjusted my distance from the wall, but my legs still feel tight. What should I do?

To reduce the tightness in your legs, you can modify the pose by bending your knees and placing your feet flat on the wall. This modification is also useful if your head, neck or back feels strained.

How can I modify the pose to help open my hips and groin?

You can change the position of your feet to perform a supported Bound Angle Pose. When your legs are up on the wall, bend your legs and place the soles of your feet together. Then slide your heels down the wall toward the floor. Only bring your heels down as far as is comfortable for you. For more information on Bound Angle Pose, see page 76.

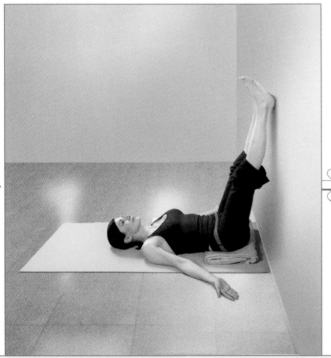

4 Place your arms on the floor a comfortable distance away from your body, with your palms facing up.

• Your shoulders and arms should be relaxed.

5 Exhale as you relax your head, neck and spine toward the floor.

6 Hold the pose for 5 to 15 minutes.

7 To come out of the pose, bend your knees and place your feet on the wall. Then roll onto your right side. Lie on your right side until you are ready to return to a seated position.

half shoulderstand *(ardha sarvangasana)*

Half Shoulderstand provides an intense stretch to your neck and shoulders. This pose is beneficial for strengthening your entire body and improving your circulation. You can also perform Half Shoulderstand to calm and rejuvenate your mind. The calmness this pose encourages can relieve insomnia, depression and mental exhaustion.

If you have trouble moving into Half Shoulderstand, you can perform Spinal Rocking to move into the pose. Once you move into the pose, try to position your body so it does not require a lot of effort to balance your legs directly above your head.

Performing Half Shoulderstand is an excellent way to prepare for Shoulderstand. Make sure you are comfortable performing Half Shoulderstand before you attempt Shoulderstand. If you are not comfortable performing Half Shoulderstand, you can try Legs Up the Wall Pose, which is less advanced and provides similar benefits.

You should avoid Half Shoulderstand if you have a neck injury, high blood pressure or if you are menstruating. You should also avoid this pose if you have an eye problem, such as glaucoma.

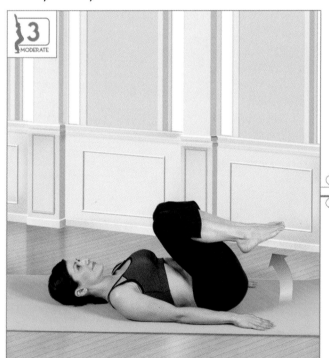

3 MODERATE

1 Lie on your back with your knees bent and the soles of your feet flat on the floor. Your feet should be together.

2 Place your arms alongside your body, with your palms facing the floor.

3 Draw your knees toward your chest.

4 Press your palms into the floor.

5 Lift your hips off the floor.

• If you have difficulty lifting your hips off the floor, you can use a rocking motion to help you.

Can I use a wall for support in this pose?

You can perform the following variation, using a wall for support. Lie on your back with the soles of your feet flat on a wall and your knees bent at a 90-degree angle. With your arms alongside your body, press your palms into the floor. Then push your feet into the wall and lift your hips off the floor. Bend your elbows, place your hands on your lower back and extend one foot above your head. Then repeat these steps, extending your other foot above your head.

What should I do if I have trouble balancing my legs in this pose?

Perform the pose as described in the steps below, except lie with your head an arm's length away from a wall. When you straighten your legs in the pose, gently rest your toes against the wall to help you balance your legs.

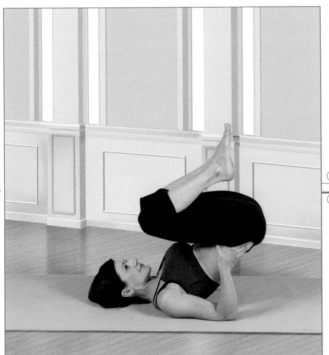

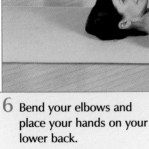

6 Bend your elbows and place your hands on your lower back.

• Your hips should be cradled in your palms.

7 Press your elbows and your upper arms into the floor to support your body.

8 Straighten your legs to position your legs at a 45-degree angle above your torso.

• Your feet should be directly above your head. Your legs should be straight, but your knees should not be locked.

9 Relax your neck.

10 Hold the pose for 30 seconds to 3 minutes. Then bring your hands to the floor with your palms facing down and slowly roll your spine down to the floor.

shoulderstand

(sarvangasana)

Shoulderstand strengthens your entire body, while stimulating your spine and thyroid gland. Your thyroid gland, located at the front of your neck, is responsible for regulating many of your bodily functions, such as your metabolism and body temperature. Performing this pose also provides a calm energy that nourishes your body and soul.

While performing Shoulderstand, make sure you do not turn your head to the side. You should also make sure that you keep your legs together without tensing your calves or feet.

If you find you are straining to hold Shoulderstand, you should come out of the pose and then try moving into the pose again. If this pose is still too difficult, you should perform an easier pose, such as Half Shoulderstand or Legs Up the Wall Pose, which can help you build the strength required for Shoulderstand.

Avoid performing Shoulderstand if you have eye, neck or shoulder problems, high or low blood pressure or heart problems. You should also avoid this pose if you are menstruating.

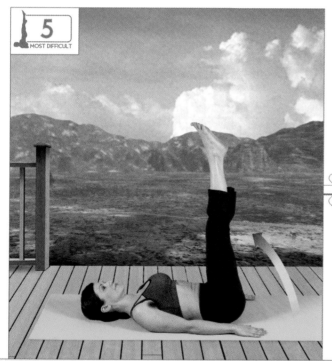

5 MOST DIFFICULT

1 Lie on your back with your legs extended and your feet together.

2 Place your arms alongside your body, with your palms facing down. Extend through your fingertips to lengthen your arms.

3 Press your palms into the floor and then raise both feet toward the ceiling to form a 90-degree angle with your body and legs.

4 Lift your hips and lower back off the floor.

5 Bend your elbows and place your hands on your lower back.

6 Press your elbows and your upper arms into the floor to support your body.

What should I do if my legs lean to one side in Shoulderstand?

Bend your knees and bring them in toward your chest. Then align your waist with your chest before straightening your legs once again.

What should I do if my chest feels heavy and I find it difficult to breathe?

Your torso may be tilting forward in the pose. To remedy this problem, push your body up through your waist, hips and thighs, keeping your buttocks in line with your body.

Can I stretch my inner thighs and hips in this pose?

Once you feel comfortable performing Shoulderstand, you can perform the following modifications while holding the pose. To stretch your inner thighs, move your legs in a scissor motion from front to back. To stretch your inner thighs and hips at the same time, bring the soles of your feet together as in Bound Angle Pose. For information on Bound Angle Pose, see page 76.

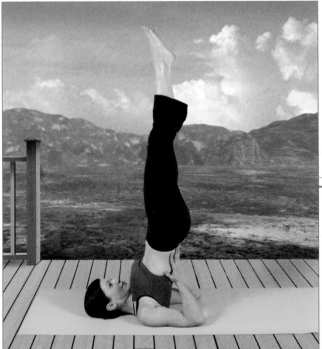

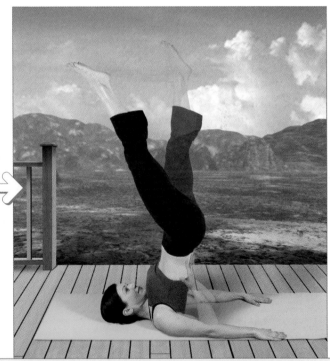

7 Move your shoulder blades together and bring your elbows as close together as possible.

8 Walk your hands up your back toward your shoulder blades, gently pushing your body up.

9 Straighten your back as much as possible.

• Your legs should be straight, but your knees should not be locked.

10 Relax your neck and shoulders.

11 Hold the pose for 30 seconds to 3 minutes.

12 To come out of the pose, lower your legs to a 45-degree angle over your head, place your palms on the floor and then slowly roll your spine down to the floor.

• After performing Shoulderstand, you should perform Fish Pose as a counter pose.

plow pose *(halasana)*

Plow Pose stretches and increases the flexibility of your spine, while providing an intense stretch for your neck. This pose also stretches the entire back of your body and stimulates the nerves in your spine. You may also want to perform this pose to calm, focus and rejuvenate your mind.

As you perform Plow Pose, make sure you do not turn your head to the side. Your head should remain in a neutral position. If you want to stretch your inner thighs in this pose, you can perform Plow Pose with

your legs spread as wide as is comfortable for you. After performing Plow Pose, you should perform a counter pose that stretches your spine in the opposite direction, such as Fish Pose.

Use caution performing Plow Pose if you have neck or shoulder problems, high or low blood pressure or heart problems. You should avoid this pose if you are menstruating or if you have eye problems, such as glaucoma.

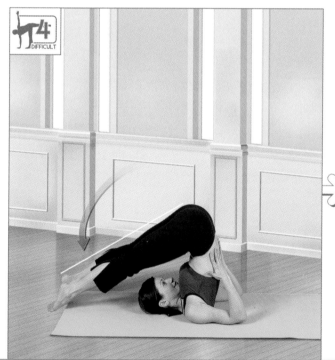

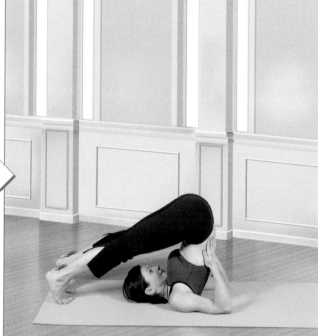

1 Begin in Shoulderstand. For information on Shoulderstand, see page 222.

2 Exhale as you slowly lower your feet toward the floor behind your head.

• Your legs should be straight, but your knees should not be locked.

• Make sure you keep your torso straight and long.

3 Flex your feet and place your toes on the floor behind your head.

4 Press your heels away from your body to lengthen your legs.

Is there an exercise I can perform to prepare for Plow Pose?

Begin in Shoulderstand and then exhale as you lower your right leg toward the floor behind your head. Then inhale as you raise your right leg. Repeat this exercise for your left leg. Then exhale as you lower both legs at the same time to move into the pose.

How can I stretch my arms and shoulders in Plow Pose?

Once your arms and hands are on the floor, interlace your fingers and stretch out through your hands. You can also try stretching your arms above your head to reach for your toes. If possible, clasp your toes in your hands.

I have difficulty performing Shoulderstand. Is there another way to move into Plow Pose?

Yes. You can gently move from Spinal Rocking into Plow Pose. For information on Spinal Rocking, see page 50.

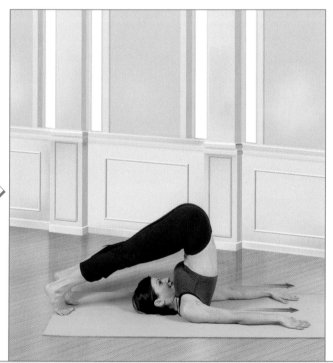

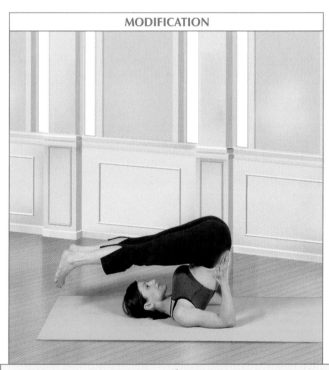

MODIFICATION

5 Place your arms on the floor, palms facing down.

6 Extend through your fingertips to lengthen your arms.

7 Hold the pose for 30 seconds to 2 minutes. Then place your hands on your lower back and return to Shoulderstand.

• If you cannot place your toes on the floor behind your head, you should keep your hands on your lower back to support your body.

1 Perform steps 1 and 2 on page 224 and then bend your elbows and place your hands on your lower back to support your body.

Chapter 13

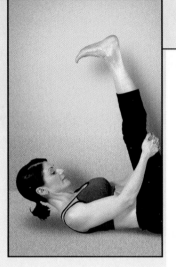

Reclined poses are usually less physically demanding than other poses. Performing certain reclined poses can improve your circulation and stretch your legs, which makes these poses especially useful as warm-up poses for forward bends that involve intense leg stretches. You may also find reclined poses relaxing as they help to relieve tension in your mind and body. This chapter takes you through several reclined poses you can incorporate into your yoga practice.

Reclined Poses

In this Chapter...

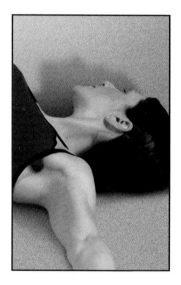

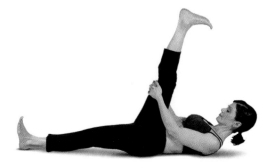

reclined
leg stretch *(supta padangusthasana)*

Reclined Leg Stretch is an excellent pose for stretching your hips, groin, hamstrings, calves and ankles. This pose can also strengthen your legs, relieve tension in your lower back and improve the circulation in your legs. You may find this pose useful to warm up your hamstrings before performing forward bends.

If you are a beginner, you can loop a yoga strap around your foot to perform Reclined Leg Stretch. If you do not have a yoga strap, you can use any cloth strap, such as a bathrobe belt. Make sure you do not hold

the strap too tightly. You should only use the strap to support your raised leg.

While performing this pose, focus on pressing the hip of your raised leg into the floor and lifting your raised heel up toward the ceiling, as you visualize your raised leg lengthening.

If you have high blood pressure, you should rest your head on a folded blanket. Make sure you use caution performing this pose if you have problems with your hips or legs.

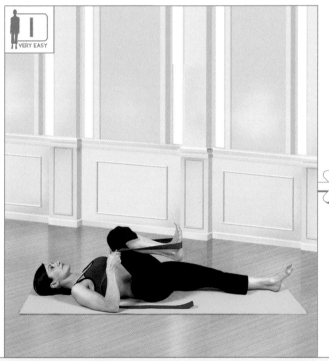

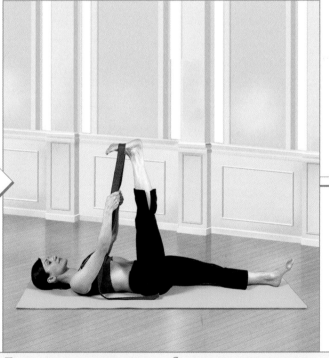

1 Lie on your back with your legs flat on the floor and your feet hip width apart.

2 Bend your right leg and draw your knee toward your chest. Keep your left leg straight and flat on the floor.

3 Loop a strap around the arch of your right foot and hold an end of the strap in each hand.

4 Relax your arms and shoulders. Keep your head and shoulders on the floor throughout the pose.

5 Inhale as you straighten your right leg, lifting your heel toward the ceiling. Press your left leg into the floor.

6 Press your right hip into the floor and your right heel toward the ceiling. Then flex your right foot and gently stretch your toes toward your body.

• Make sure both your legs are straight, but your knees are not locked.

How can I vary Reclined Leg Stretch?

Perform the pose as described below, except lower your raised leg to the side until you feel a comfortable stretch in your inner thigh. Then raise your leg back up until it is perpendicular to the floor. You can also cross your raised leg to the opposite side of your body and then raise it back up until it is perpendicular to the floor. You should hold your leg in each position for an equal length of time, making sure both of your hips remain in contact with the floor. These variations strengthen your pelvis and open your hips.

How can I deepen the pose?

To deepen the pose, perform the pose as described below, except without a yoga strap. Instead, grip the big toe of your raised foot using the hand on the same side as your raised leg. Use your index, middle fingers and thumb to grip your big toe. This variation requires a great deal of flexibility.

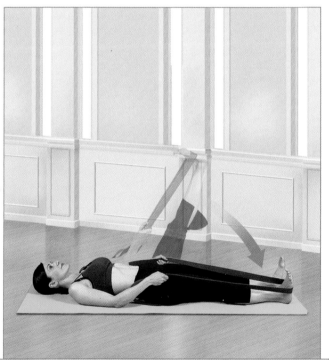

MODIFICATION

7 Hold the pose for 30 seconds to 1 minute.

8 To come out of the pose, exhale as you lower your leg back to the floor, keeping your leg straight.

9 Repeat steps **1** to **8** for your other side.

• If you have lower back problems or you find it difficult to straighten your leg, you can perform Reclined Leg Stretch with one knee bent.

1 Perform Reclined Leg Stretch, except bend your left leg and place the bottom of your left foot flat on the floor.

reclined head to knee pose

Reclined Head to Knee Pose stretches your hamstrings, while improving the circulation in your legs. This pose also increases the flexibility of your pelvic area and stimulates your abdominals, which helps to improve digestion and elimination. You can also use this pose to strengthen and relieve stiffness in your lower back.

You may want to perform Reclined Head to Knee Pose to warm up for forward bends, such as Seated Forward Bend and Standing Wide Angle Forward Bend. This pose is a good warm-up pose for forward bends

because it helps prepare your hamstrings for the intense stretch involved in forward bends.

As you bring your forehead toward your knee in this pose, make sure you also lift your chest toward your thigh, otherwise you may strain your neck. Also, you should bring your forehead and knee only as close together as is comfortable for you.

Make sure you use caution performing Reclined Head to Knee Pose if you have lower back or neck problems.

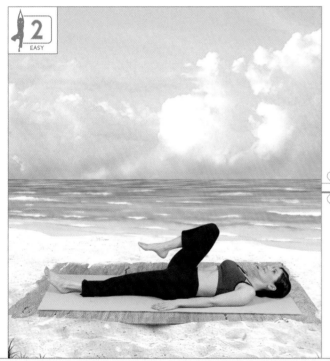
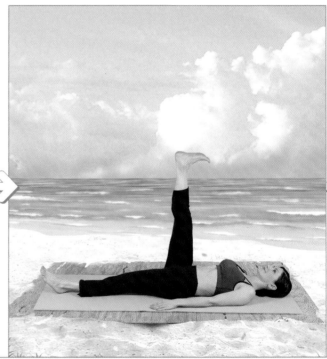

1 Lie on your back with your legs extended and your feet together.

2 Place your arms on the floor at your sides, with your palms facing down.

3 Bend your right leg and draw your right knee toward your chest.

• Keep your left leg straight and flat on the floor.

4 Press your lower back into the floor.

5 Straighten your right leg above you.

• Make sure your right knee is not locked.

My lower back feels strained in this pose. What can I do?

Before you raise your leg in this pose, you can bend your other leg and place the sole of your foot on the floor, instead of leaving your leg straight and flat on the floor.

How can I modify the pose if my neck feels strained?

If your neck feels strained when you bring your forehead toward your knee, you should keep your head on the floor throughout the pose.

What should I do if resting my head on the floor is uncomfortable?

If your head does not rest comfortably on the floor, place a folded blanket or towel under your head, neck and shoulders. This modification is also useful if you have high blood pressure, since the blanket allows you to position your head above your heart.

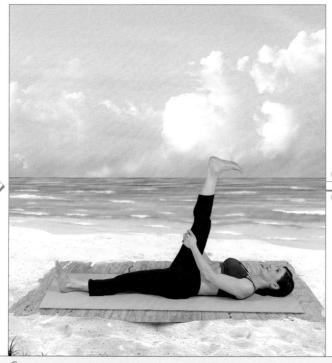

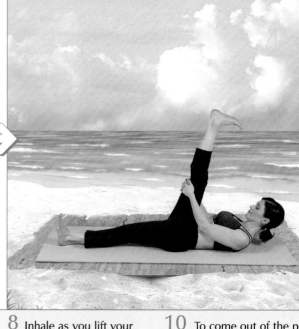

6 Interlace your fingers behind your right thigh.

7 Gently pull your right leg toward your body.

• Keep your arms and shoulders relaxed.

8 Inhale as you lift your chest toward your right thigh and bring your forehead toward your right knee, keeping your neck relaxed.

9 Hold the pose for 15 to 30 seconds.

10 To come out of the pose, exhale as you lower your head, neck and shoulders back to the floor. Then release your hands and lower your leg.

11 Repeat steps 3 to 10 for your other side.

raised knee to chest pose

Raised Knee to Chest Pose is a great pose for strengthening your abdominals and lower back. By stimulating your abdominal area, this pose can also help improve digestion and elimination. Regular practice of this pose can improve the flexibility in your hips.

As you lift your upper body toward your knee in this pose, make sure that you lift your chest, not just your head, to avoid straining your neck. You should also make sure you do not round your shoulders forward when you lift your upper body. Your chest should remain open and your neck and shoulders should be as relaxed as possible.

Since this pose can be strenuous, you may have a tendency to hold your breath while performing the pose. It is important to remember to breathe evenly as you hold this pose, allowing your breath to energize your body.

Make sure you use caution performing Raised Knee to Chest Pose if you have problems with your neck, lower back or knees.

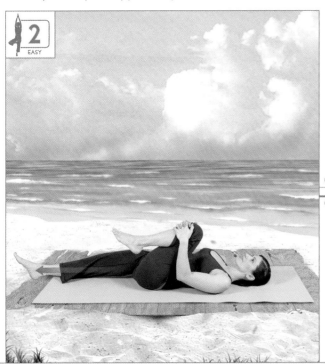

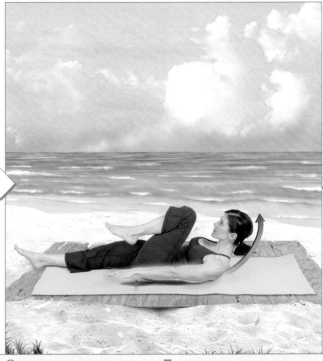

1 Begin in Little Boat Pose. For information on Little Boat Pose, see page 58.

2 Extend your right leg along the floor.

• Keep your right leg straight, but make sure your right knee is not locked.

• Keep your left knee bent into your chest.

3 Extend your arms alongside your body with your palms facing down.

4 Exhale as you press your lower back into the floor.

5 Inhale as you lift your upper body toward your left knee, allowing your arms to rise slightly off the floor.

• Make sure you keep your shoulders relaxed and down and keep your chest open.

What should I do if my lower back feels strained in this pose?

Perform the pose as described in the steps below, except keep both knees bent into your chest as you lift your upper body toward your knees and lift and extend your arms. This modification helps you keep your lower back pressed into the floor, which helps to protect your lower back from strain.

How can I make Raised Knee to Chest Pose easier?

Instead of raising your extended leg off the floor, you can leave this leg on the floor. If you still find the pose difficult, bend your extended leg and place the sole of your foot flat on the floor. These modifications make the pose easier on your lower back and abdominals. You can practice the pose with either of these modifications until you build up the strength required by your abdominals to perform the full version of the pose.

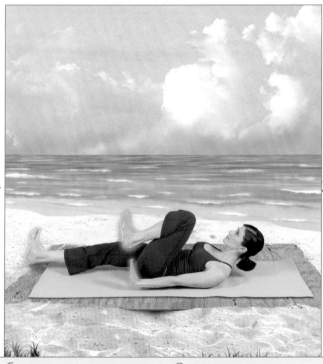

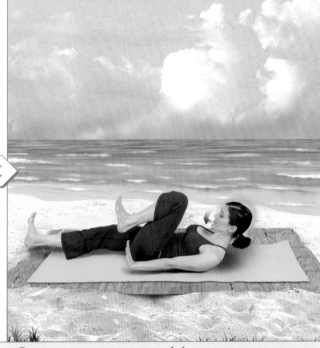

6 Flex your wrists and point your fingers toward the ceiling.

7 Flex both feet and point your toes toward the ceiling.

8 Inhale as you raise your right leg slightly off the floor.

9 Tuck your chin toward your chest and look forward.

10 Hold the pose for 5 to 30 seconds.

11 To come out of the pose, exhale as you lower your right leg, upper body and head back down to the floor and return to Little Boat Pose.

12 Repeat steps 2 to 11 for your other side.

reclined thigh-over-thigh
twist *(supta parivartanasana)*

Reclined Thigh-Over-Thigh Twist can relieve tension in your spine and hips by twisting your spine and stretching your hips. This pose also helps to open your chest, shoulders and lower back. As you twist in this pose, you massage your abdominal organs, which helps to improve digestion and elimination.

If you are having difficulty sleeping, you can perform this pose to help calm your mind and relax your body for sleep. You should feel calm and rejuvenated after

performing Reclined Thigh-Over-Thigh Twist.

If you find your arms and shoulders tend to lift off the floor as you move into the twist, focus on pressing your arms and shoulders back down to the floor. As you hold Reclined Thigh-Over-Thigh Twist, remember to breathe evenly, allowing your body to soften and release further into the twist with each exhalation.

You should be careful performing this pose if you have a hip injury or problems with your spine.

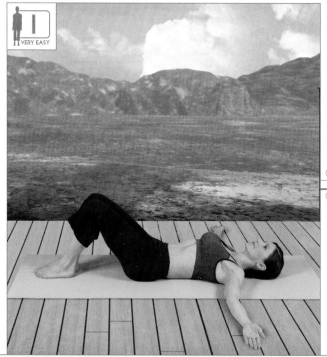

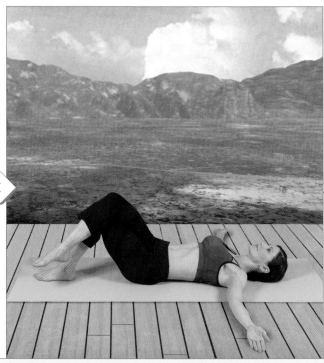

1 Lie on your back with your knees bent and your feet together. The soles of your feet should be flat on the floor.

2 Rest your arms out to your sides at shoulder height, with your palms facing up.

3 Cross your right leg over your left thigh.

• Make sure there is no space between your thighs.

My neck feels strained when I turn my head to look at my hand. What should I do?

If your neck feels strained, you can look up at the ceiling and tilt your chin down slightly to lengthen the back of your neck.

How can I deepen the pose?

While holding the pose, place the hand closest to your knee on your thigh and gently press your leg closer toward the floor. Make sure you do not pull on your leg.

How can I modify the pose to stretch my hips more?

Perform steps **1** to **2** below and then cross your right ankle over your left thigh so that your right shin is parallel to the floor. Then lower your left knee so that the sole of your right foot comes to rest on the floor. After holding the pose for 15 to 45 seconds, repeat these steps for your other side.

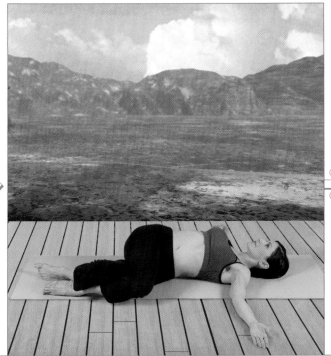

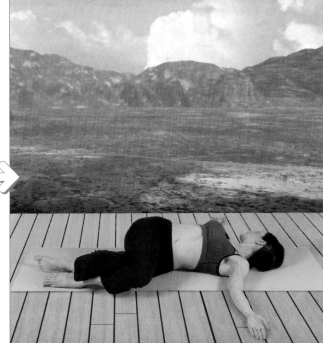

4 Exhale as you lower your knees toward the floor on the left side of your body.

• Allow your knees to drop until you feel a comfortable stretch. Your knees do not have to rest on the floor.

5 Turn your head to look at your right hand.

6 Hold the pose for 15 to 45 seconds and then inhale as you bring your knees back to the center and rest your feet on the floor.

7 Repeat steps **3** to **6** for your other side.

knee down
twist *(supta matsyendrasana)*

Knee Down Twist improves the flexibility of your spine. Performing this pose also opens your chest and shoulders, while stretching your lower back and hips.

You may find Knee Down Twist useful for releasing tension in your spine, hips and abdomen. This pose can also relax your nervous system and calm your mind. If you have difficulty sleeping, you may want to perform Knee Down Twist to relax your body and mind before going to sleep.

As you perform Knee Down Twist, only lower your knee as far as is comfortable for you. It is more important to keep both of your shoulders on the floor than to lower your knee all the way to the floor. As you hold the pose, allow your body to soften and release further into the twist with each exhalation.

You should use caution performing Knee Down Twist if you have problems with your spine, lower back, hips or knees.

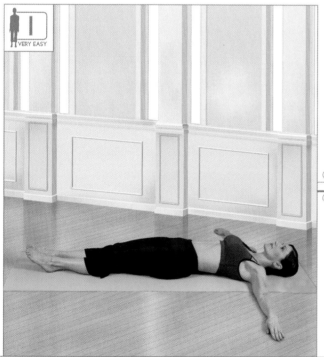

VERY EASY

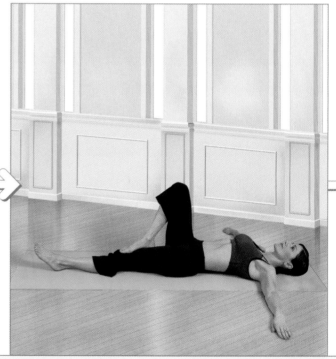

1 Lie on your back with your legs extended and your feet together.

2 Place your arms on the floor out to your sides at shoulder height, with your palms facing down.

3 Press out through the crown of your head, fingertips and toes to lengthen your entire body.

4 Bend your right leg.

5 Place the sole of your right foot on top of your left leg, just above your left knee.

When I move into the twist, my shoulder lifts off the floor. What should I do?

As you move into the pose, you can let your shoulder lift off the floor. You should then use your breath to encourage your shoulder to move back down toward the floor. With each exhalation, allow your shoulder to soften and release back down toward the floor.

What can I do if my neck feels strained in this pose?

Instead of looking over your shoulder, you can look up at the ceiling and tilt your chin down slightly to lengthen the back of your neck.

How can I keep my leg stable in this pose?

As you hold the pose, place the hand closest to your bent knee on your knee to keep your leg stable. Make sure you do not pull your knee toward the floor.

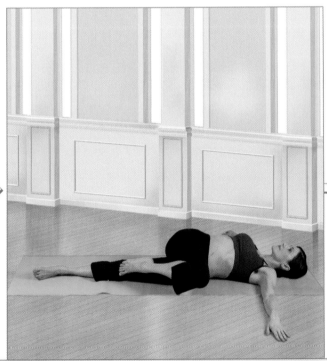

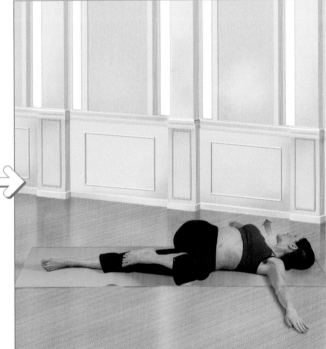

6 Exhale as you lower your right knee toward the floor on the left side of your body.

• Allow your knee to lower until you feel a comfortable stretch. Your knee does not have to rest on the floor.

• Make sure your shoulders and arms are relaxed down on the floor.

7 Turn your head to look over your right shoulder.

8 Hold the pose for 20 seconds to 1 minute.

9 To come out of the pose, inhale as you bring your right knee and head back to the center and then extend your right leg on the floor.

10 Repeat steps 4 to 9 for your other side.

reclined bound angle pose *(supta baddha konasana)*

Reclined Bound Angle Pose is a restful pose that helps to open your hips and pelvis. This pose also provides a good stretch to your groin and inner thighs.

You can easily increase or decrease the intensity of the stretch in this pose by changing the position of your feet. The closer your feet are to your groin, the greater the intensity of the stretch. The further your feet are away from your groin, the lower the intensity of the stretch.

For extra support in this pose, you can place a folded blanket under your head and upper back. You can also place a folded blanket under your lower back if your lower back lifts off the floor.

To modify this pose, you can keep one leg extended. You can also place a folded blanket under the thigh of your bent leg to support your knee in this modification.

Use caution performing this pose if you have a knee, hip, lower back or groin injury.

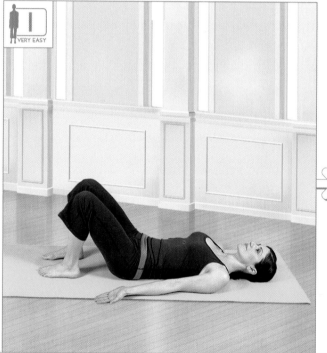

VERY EASY

1 Begin in Relaxation Pose. For information on Relaxation Pose, see page 242.

2 Lay your arms at your sides on the floor, with your palms facing up.

3 Bend your knees and place the soles of your feet flat on the floor.

4 Bring the soles of your feet together and allow your knees to drop toward the floor.

5 Move your heels toward your groin as far as is comfortable for you.

• The closer your heels are to your groin, the more intense the stretch will be.

What should I do if my hips are stiff in this pose?

You can place folded blankets under each thigh to support your knees. This allows your hips to release so your knees drop down into the blankets as far as possible.

How can I stretch my shoulders in this pose?

To stretch your shoulders, place your arms on the floor above your head with your palms facing the ceiling. This also opens your chest to improve your capacity for deep breathing.

How can I reduce the strain in my inner thighs and groin?

To reduce the strain in your inner thighs and groin, perform the pose with your feet on a prop, such as a padded block or bolster. You can experiment with the height of the prop to determine what height feels the most comfortable for you.

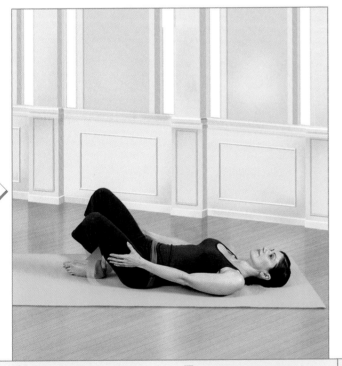

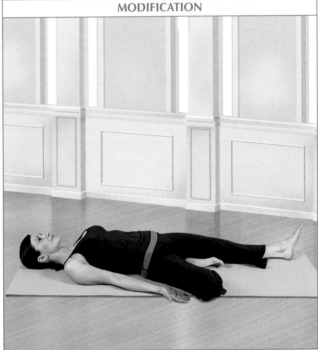

MODIFICATION

6 Hold the pose for 30 seconds to 1 minute.

7 To come out of the pose, use your hands to press your thighs together, then roll over onto one side and move to a seated position.

• You can perform Reclined Bound Angle Pose while keeping one leg extended.

1 Begin in Relaxation Pose and then bend your right knee.

2 Place the sole of your right foot on the inside of your left leg, as close to your groin as is comfortable.

3 Hold the pose for 30 seconds to 1 minute and then switch legs.

Chapter 14

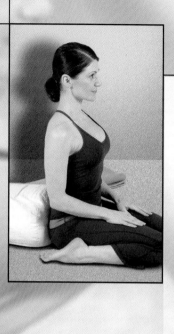

You should always leave time for performing a relaxation or restorative pose at the end of your yoga practice. Restorative poses, such as Supported Reclining Hero Pose, involve props, such as bolsters or blankets, to enhance relaxation. Restorative and relaxation poses are also good to practice during times of illness or when you feel low on energy. This chapter teaches you relaxation and restorative poses that will allow you to end your yoga practice feeling calm and rejuvenated.

Relaxation and Restorative Poses

In this Chapter...

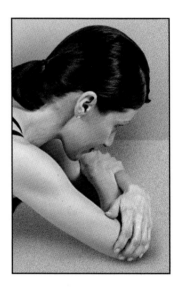

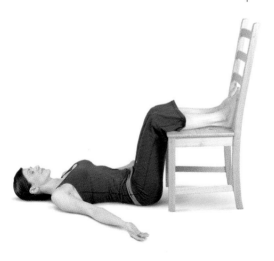

relaxation pose *(savasana)*

Relaxation Pose is a resting pose that helps you feel aware, rejuvenated and free from tension. You may find this pose useful for relaxing your mind and body. It is important to perform this pose at the end of each yoga practice.

Performing Relaxation Pose can help relieve stress and mild depression. This pose can also help reduce ailments such as headaches, fatigue and insomnia.

While performing this pose, you should think about relaxing each part of your body individually, from your head down to your feet. To help yourself relax, focus on your breathing, especially on exhaling as you relax your body to the floor. When your mind wanders to other thoughts, bring your attention back to your breath and body. If you perform the pose for several minutes, you may want to cover your body with a blanket, since your body temperature may drop.

If you have back problems, you should place a prop under your knees or put your calves up on the seat of a chair.

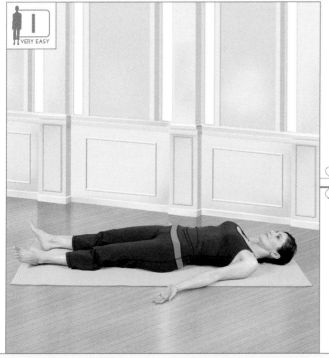

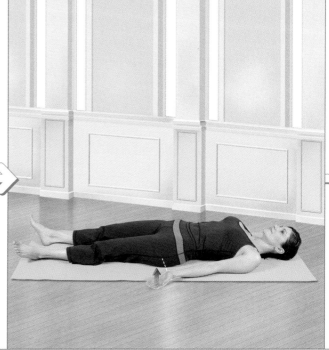

1 Lie on your back with your legs flat on the floor and your feet hip to shoulder width apart.

- Make sure your spine is straight and your head is in line with your spine.

2 Exhale as you relax your legs and feet and allow them to turn out to the sides.

3 Lay your arms down along the sides of your body and place your hands on the floor 6 to 8 inches away from your hips, with your palms facing up.

4 Exhale as you relax your shoulders down to the floor and relax your arms away from your shoulders.

How can I make sure my head is in line with my spine?

You may find you accidentally turn or tilt your head to one side in Relaxation Pose. To make sure your head is in line with your spine, align your chin with the notch in the middle of your collar bone. You should also try to keep the back of your neck long—either by dropping your chin slightly toward your chest or by placing a folded blanket under your head. It is particularly important to keep your neck long if your neck or upper shoulders are tight.

How can I improve my relaxation in this pose?

If your eyes are active in Relaxation Pose, your mind may be active as well. To improve your relaxation, place an eye bag over your closed eyes. The weight of the eye bag can help relax your eyes and, in turn, relax your mind.

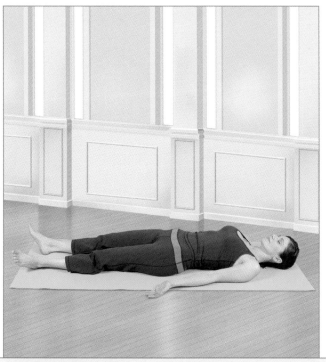

MODIFICATION

5 Close your eyes and relax your entire body, releasing any tension that you may have.

• Visualize your body melting into the floor.

6 Hold the pose for 5 to 20 minutes.

7 To come out of the pose, open your eyes, bend your right leg and then roll onto your right side. Press your hands into the floor as you slowly come up to a sitting position.

• If you have lower back problems, you should perform Relaxation Pose with your knees bent to reduce the strain on your lower back.

1 Perform Relaxation Pose, except place a pillow, bolster or rolled blanket under your knees. You can also place your calves on the seat of a chair as shown above.

crocodile pose *(makarasana)*

Crocodile Pose is a passive back bend that is useful for relieving stress and tension in your body. This pose also helps to regulate your blood pressure, improve digestion and relax your body for sleep. You should feel calm and rejuvenated after performing Crocodile Pose.

Since this pose massages the uterus, women can use the pose to relieve severe menstrual cramps. You can also use this pose to help alleviate pain in your neck and jaw.

This pose is a good alternative to Relaxation Pose, especially if you find it difficult to relax while lying on your back. You may want to perform this pose at the beginning or end of your practice, or between more intense back bends, such as Cobra Pose and Bow Pose.

Remember to breathe deeply in this pose to help release tension in your entire body, especially your lower back. As you inhale, feel your back gently rise and expand. As you exhale, feel your back softly release toward the floor.

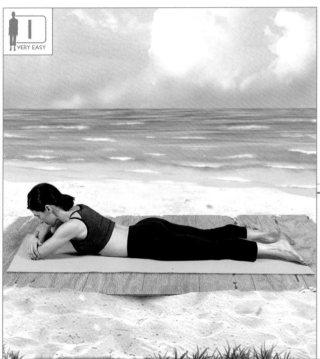

VERY EASY

1 Lie face down with your legs extended behind you a comfortable distance apart.

- The top of your feet should be resting on the floor and your toes should be pointing outward.

2 Cross your arms in front of your head and rest the palm of each hand on the opposite elbow.

3 Draw your elbows toward your body slightly to raise your shoulders and upper chest slightly off the floor.

4 Bow your head and rest your forehead on your forearms.

- Make sure your neck and shoulders remain relaxed.

5 Close your eyes and let your entire body relax into the floor.

6 Hold the pose for 30 seconds to 3 minutes.

- Breathe deeply and notice how your stomach presses into the floor with each inhalation.

My shoulders are uncomfortable in this pose. What can I do?

You can place your arms in a position that is more relaxing for your shoulders. Rest your arms on the floor above your head with your elbows bent so your forearms form a comfortable angle. Place one hand on top of the other and then gently rest your chin or forehead on the floor.

Is there another way to vary Crocodile Pose?

Yes. Instead of crossing your arms in this pose, bend your elbows and place one hand on top of the other to make a pillow for your head. Then turn your head and rest one cheek on your hands as you hold the pose. Then turn your head, rest your other cheek on your hands and hold the pose. You may find this position more comfortable than resting your forehead on your forearms.

MODIFICATION 1

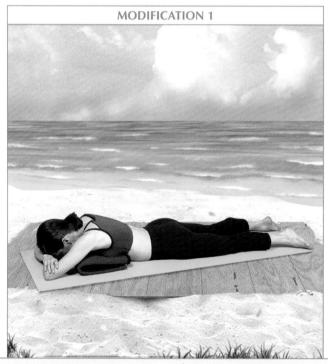

MODIFICATION 2

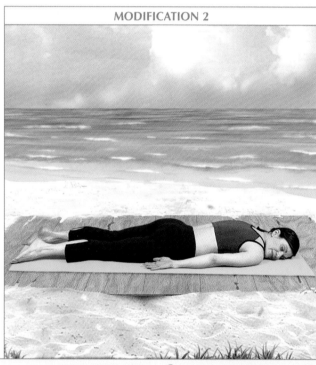

• You can use a prop to make Crocodile Pose easier on your shoulders and neck. This modification also lets you breathe through your nose more easily.

1 Rest your chest on a prop, such as a thin cushion, folded blanket or towel, while you perform the pose. Your chin should hang over the edge of the prop.

• You can perform a more restful variation of Crocodile Pose.

1 Lie face down with your arms resting at your sides, palms up. Turn your head to the right and rest your cheek on the floor.

2 After holding the pose, turn your head to the left and rest your other cheek on the floor for the same amount of time.

supported reclining
hero pose *(supta virasana)*

Supported Reclining Hero Pose opens your chest and rib cage, which helps to relieve breathing problems and can be beneficial for your heart. This pose also alleviates sinus pressure, reduces fatigue in your legs and relieves nausea and indigestion. If you are feeling stressed or anxious, you may want to perform this pose to soothe your mind and relax your nervous system.

Supported Reclining Hero Pose requires the use of props, which allows you to hold the pose for a longer period of time. The bolster used in this pose prevents

your knees from coming off the floor and also helps to lift and stretch your torso and chest. The folded blanket used in this pose rests under your head so you can keep your head in alignment with your spine.

You should be comfortable sitting in Hero Pose before you attempt this pose. After performing this pose, you should shake out your legs to help relieve your knees, ankles and feet. Avoid this pose if you have knee or lower back problems.

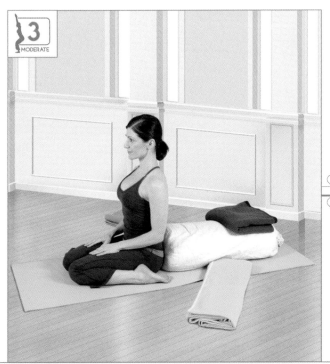

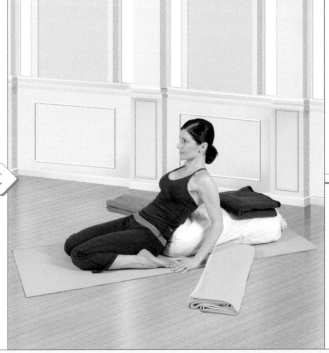

1 Place a bolster on the floor with a folded blanket on top of one end of the bolster. Then position folded blankets on either side of the bolster.

2 Sit in Hero Pose in front of the opposite end of the bolster. For information on Hero Pose, see page 92.

- The end of the bolster should touch your tailbone.

3 Press your sitting bones toward the floor and the crown of your head toward the ceiling.

4 Place your palms or fingertips on the floor beside your toes, with your fingers pointing forward.

5 Slowly bend your elbows and lean back onto the bolster.

- Make sure your knees stay on the floor.

What should I do if my lower back feels strained in this pose?

You should increase the height of the entire bolster so you do not have to lean so far back. Place thickly folded blankets on top of the bolster until you can lean back without straining your lower back.

How can I reduce the strain on my knees in this pose?

You can position a cushion between your calves and thighs behind your knees to reduce the strain.

How can I ensure I remain relaxed in this pose?

It is important to make sure you properly support your head and neck with the folded blanket at the end of the bolster. If the blanket is too thick, you may compress the front of your neck. If the blanket is too thin, you may extend your neck too far back. Adjust the blanket until you feel comfortable in the pose.

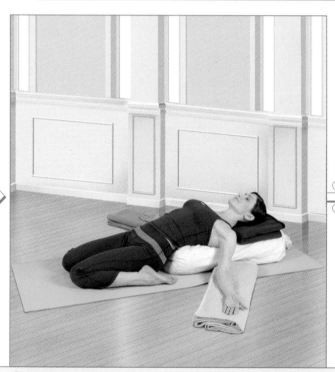

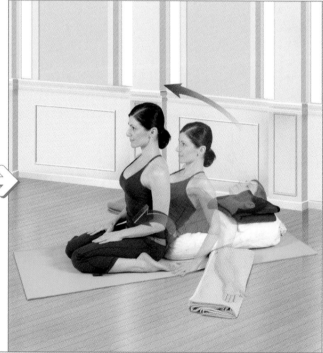

6 Rest your head on the folded blanket at the end of the bolster.

7 Lay your arms down along the sides of your body on the folded blankets.

• Your arms should be at a 45-degree angle with your body, with your palms facing up.

8 Exhale as you relax your entire body, releasing any tension that you may have.

9 Hold the pose for 1 to 3 minutes.

10 To come out of the pose, press your palms into the floor to help you lift your torso to an upright position and return to Hero Pose.

Chapter 15

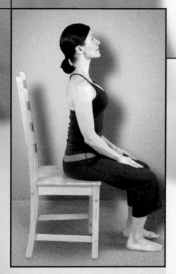

Sessions of yoga are known as yoga practices. Yoga practices should always be well balanced—including forward, backward and twisting movements of your spine—and geared to your fitness level. This chapter shows you how to create a personal yoga practice to suit your needs. You will also find numerous sample warm-up sequences and yoga practices you can perform or use as guidelines for creating your own yoga practices.

Yoga Practices

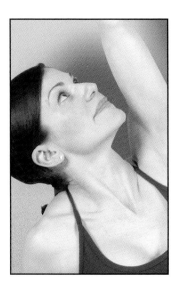

In this Chapter...

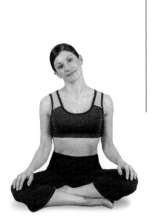

creating a personal yoga practice

You can create a personal yoga practice to meet your needs. To help you decide on which poses to perform, you may want to start with poses that you enjoy performing and then develop your practice from there. Make sure the poses you select include forward, backward and twisting movements of the spine, as well as shoulder and hip movements. You should spend an average of 2 minutes on each pose, resting between poses whenever you need to.

When you design your own yoga practice, plan to practice for 60 to 90 minutes. However, if you are short on time, you can create a shorter practice of 15 to 30 minutes. You should also make sure you adjust the intensity of your practice according to how you feel at the time.

If you have health problems, be sure to discuss practicing yoga with your doctor and seek the advice of a qualified yoga teacher before designing your personal yoga practice.

1) Centering and Breath Awareness

At the beginning of every yoga practice, you should spend 5 to 10 minutes focusing on centering and breath awareness. This time allows you to bring your attention to the present moment and prepares you for your practice. Once you are in a comfortable seated or relaxation pose, perform breathing exercises, such as the exercises shown on pages 36 to 39, and become aware of your breath and body.

2) Counter Poses

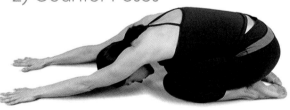

Counter poses are an important part of your yoga practice. A counter pose moves your spine in the opposite direction from the previous pose and allows your spine to return to a neutral position. Forward bends are good counter poses for back bends, twists and side bends. Gentle back bends are good counter poses for forward bends.

3) Warm Ups

You should perform a warm-up sequence to prepare your entire body for your practice. A warm-up sequence warms up your muscles, increases the flexibility in your joints and improves your circulation. You can choose to perform a seated, reclined or standing warm-up sequence, as shown on pages 252 to 257. You can also create your own warm-up sequence by performing a combination of the warm-up poses shown on pages 48 to 69 and neck, shoulder and arm stretches shown on pages 42 to 47.

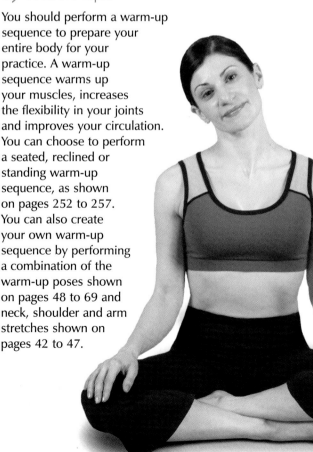

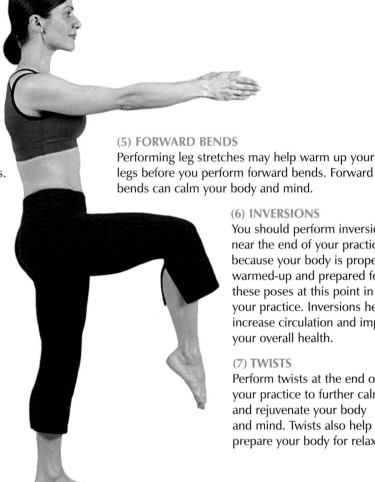

4) The Poses

You can follow these guidelines to help you develop the order of poses in your practice:

(1) SUN SALUTATION

Before beginning the poses in your practice, you may want to perform Sun Salutation, starting on page 262, to prepare for the poses.

(2) STANDING POSES

You should perform standing poses next to improve your posture, as well as energize and strengthen your entire body.

(3) BALANCING POSES

Balancing poses should follow standing poses to improve your balance and coordination. Keeping your body balanced in balancing poses also encourages you to focus your mind.

(4) BACK BENDS

Back bends, which can be intense and challenging, should be performed next. You should always perform forward bends after back bends to return your spine to a neutral position.

(5) FORWARD BENDS

Performing leg stretches may help warm up your legs before you perform forward bends. Forward bends can calm your body and mind.

(6) INVERSIONS

You should perform inversions near the end of your practice because your body is properly warmed-up and prepared for these poses at this point in your practice. Inversions help increase circulation and improve your overall health.

(7) TWISTS

Perform twists at the end of your practice to further calm and rejuvenate your body and mind. Twists also help prepare your body for relaxation.

5) Relaxation

Your relaxation period should be between 5 and 15 minutes, depending on the length of your practice. Position yourself in Relaxation Pose, as shown on page 242, and allow your mind and body to relax.

Even if your practice is short, you should allow time for relaxation at the end of your practice. You should always end your yoga practice feeling relaxed and rejuvenated.

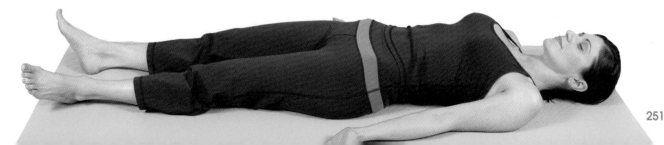

seated
warm-up sequence

You can perform Seated Warm-Up Sequence to prepare your entire body for a yoga session. This sequence warms up your muscles, increases the flexibility of your joints and gets your blood circulating. This sequence can also loosen stiff muscles to prevent injury.

You should perform a warm-up sequence, such as Seated Warm-Up Sequence, at the start of every yoga session. If you are performing a long yoga session, you should perform a longer warm-up sequence. If you are a beginner, you may also need to spend more time warming up.

SEATED WARM-UP SEQUENCE

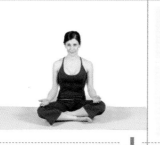

1 Begin in Easy Pose.

- For information on Easy Pose, see page 74.

2 Press your sitting bones toward the floor and point the crown of your head toward the ceiling to lengthen your spine.

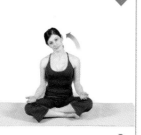

3 Perform neck stretches to relax your head and warm up your neck.

- For information on neck stretches, see page 42.

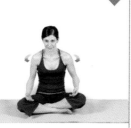

4 Perform shoulder stretches to relieve tightness and tension in your upper back and shoulders.

- For information on shoulder stretches, see page 44.

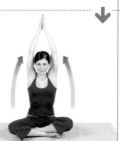

5 Perform arm stretches to warm up your arms and improve circulation in your upper body.

- For information on arm stretches, see page 46.

SEATED WARM-UP SEQUENCE (CONTINUED)

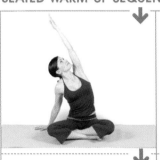

6 Place your right palm on the floor beside your right hip and raise your left arm overhead.

7 Stretch to the right to move into Seated Side Bend and stretch the side of your body.

- For information on Seated Side Bend, see page 82.

8 Perform Seated Side Bend for your other side and then return to Easy Pose.

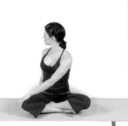

9 Turn your upper body toward the right and move into Simple Twist.

- For information on Simple Twist, see page 84.

- Simple Twist helps to increase the flexibility of your spine and upper back.

10 Perform Simple Twist for your other side and then return to Easy Pose.

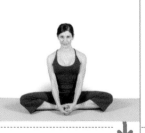

11 Bring the soles of your feet together in front of you to move into Bound Angle Pose.

- For information on Bound Angle Pose, see page 76.

- Bound Angle Pose provides a stretch to your groin and inner thighs.

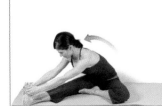

12 Extend your right leg on a diagonal and raise your arms above your head with your palms facing in.

13 Bend forward from your hips over your right leg to move into Head to Knee Pose.

- For information on Head to Knee Pose, see page 98.

- Head to Knee Pose stretches the back of your legs.

14 Repeat Head to Knee Pose for your other side and then return to Easy Pose.

reclined
warm-up sequence

You can perform Reclined Warm-Up Sequence to prepare your entire body for a yoga session. This sequence increases your blood circulation, warms up your muscles and increases the flexibility of your joints. Reclined Warm-Up Sequence can also soothe your nervous system and rejuvenate your mind.

You should perform a warm-up sequence, such as Reclined Warm-Up Sequence, at the start of every yoga session. If you are a beginner or planning a long yoga session, you should perform a longer warm-up sequence.

RECLINED WARM-UP SEQUENCE

1 Begin in Relaxation Pose.

- For information on Relaxation Pose, see page 242.

2 Relax your shoulders down to the floor and relax your arms away from your shoulders.

3 Exhale as you gently roll your head to your right side.

4 Inhale as you roll your head back to the center.

5 Exhale as you gently roll your head to your left side.

6 Inhale as your roll your head back to the center.

7 Repeat steps 3 to 6 three to five times.

- Rolling your head relaxes your head and warms up your neck.

8 Bring your knees into your chest and move into Little Boat Pose to prepare for Windmill Pose.

- For information on Little Boat Pose, see page 58.

9 Perform Windmill Pose to stretch your arms, legs and the sides of your body.

- For information on Windmill Pose, see page 62.

10 Bend your knees and place your feet flat on the floor with your heels directly under your knees.

11 Perform Pelvic Tilt to warm up your lower back and pelvis.

- For information on Pelvic Tilt, see page 56.

RECLINED WARM-UP SEQUENCE (CONTINUED)

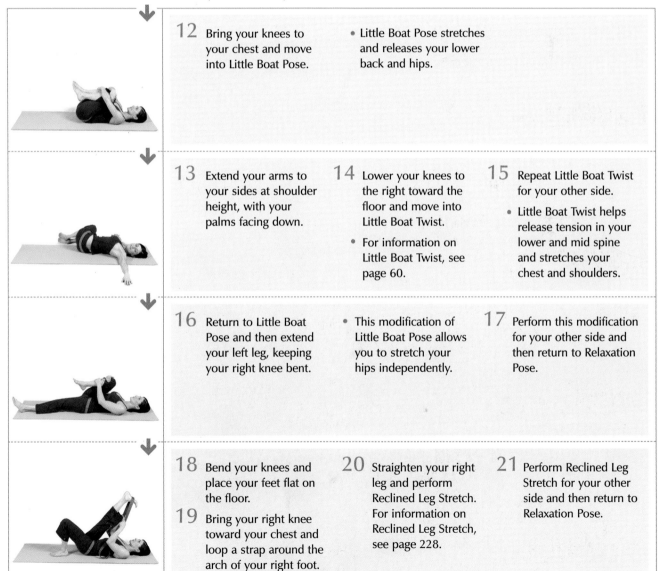

12 Bring your knees to your chest and move into Little Boat Pose.

- Little Boat Pose stretches and releases your lower back and hips.

13 Extend your arms to your sides at shoulder height, with your palms facing down.

14 Lower your knees to the right toward the floor and move into Little Boat Twist.

- For information on Little Boat Twist, see page 60.

15 Repeat Little Boat Twist for your other side.

- Little Boat Twist helps release tension in your lower and mid spine and stretches your chest and shoulders.

16 Return to Little Boat Pose and then extend your left leg, keeping your right knee bent.

- This modification of Little Boat Pose allows you to stretch your hips independently.

17 Perform this modification for your other side and then return to Relaxation Pose.

18 Bend your knees and place your feet flat on the floor.

19 Bring your right knee toward your chest and loop a strap around the arch of your right foot.

20 Straighten your right leg and perform Reclined Leg Stretch. For information on Reclined Leg Stretch, see page 228.

21 Perform Reclined Leg Stretch for your other side and then return to Relaxation Pose.

standing warm-up sequence

Standing Warm-Up Sequence helps to warm up your muscles, gently increase the flexibility in your joints and stimulate your circulation, preparing your entire body for your practice. By warming up your muscles, this sequence also helps to avoid injury as you perform your practice. When you stretch your muscles in this warm-up, make sure that you do not overdo it.

This sequence is an especially good warm-up for a more physically demanding practice, such as Strengthening Practice shown on page 290.

STANDING WARM-UP SEQUENCE

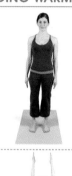

1 Begin in Mountain Pose.

- For information on Mountain Pose, see page 120.

- Your lower body should feel stable and grounded and your upper body should feel light and relaxed.

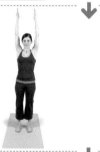

2 Raise your arms above your head, keeping your shoulders relaxed and down.

- Your arms should be shoulder width apart and your palms should be facing each other.

- This modification of Mountain Pose stretches your arms and shoulders.

3 Position your hands in Prayer Pose. For information on Prayer Pose, see page 48.

4 Circle your arms out to each side and then bring your palms together overhead to perform arm stretches.

- For information on arm stretches, see page 46.

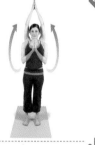

5 Place your right hand on your right hip and raise your left arm up over your head with your palm facing in.

6 Lean to the right to stretch your left side.

- This is an energizing pose that opens and stretches the sides of your body.

7 Repeat steps 5 and 6 for your other side and then return to Mountain Pose.

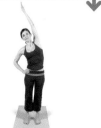

STANDING WARM-UP SEQUENCE (CONTINUED)

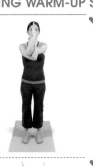

8 Raise your arms to shoulder height in front of you, palms facing up.

9 Cross your left arm over your right arm so your elbows are on top of each other.

10 Bend your elbows and wrap your forearms around each other so your palms are facing each other, with your fingers pointing toward the ceiling.

11 Lift your hands and arms up toward the ceiling.

12 Repeat steps 8 to 11 for your other side and then return to Mountain Pose.

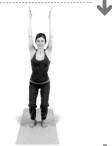

13 Raise your arms above your head, with your palms facing each other, shoulder width apart and your upper arms beside your ears.

14 Bend your knees and move into Chair Pose.

- For information on Chair Pose, see page 126.

- Chair Pose strengthens your lower body and torso.

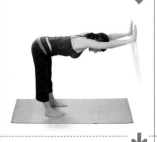

15 Stand in Mountain Pose facing a wall, with your palms on the wall at shoulder height.

16 Slowly walk backward and walk your hands down the wall to move into Right Angle Pose.

- For information on Right Angle Pose, see page 152.

- Right Angle Pose provides a deep stretch to your shoulders, arms, back and hamstrings.

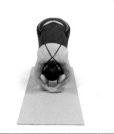

17 Move into Mountain Pose and then step your right foot to the right 2 to 3 feet.

18 Bend forward from your hips, bending your knees slightly. Then relax your head and neck toward the floor to move into Rag Doll Pose.

- For information on Rag Doll Pose, see page 168.

- Rag Doll Pose is useful for lengthening your spine and increasing the flexibility in the back of your legs.

beginner sun salutation *(surya namaskar variation)*

Beginner Sun Salutation is an easier version of Sun Salutation, which is a sequence of poses that warms up your entire body, while helping to unite your body, breath and mind.

If you only have time for a quick practice, you may want to perform this series on its own to strengthen and stretch all of your major muscle groups, while stimulating your cardiovascular system.

The poses in Beginner Sun Salutation are geared toward people with less flexibility or mobility, such as beginners and seniors.

As you perform the poses, it is important to concentrate on breathing easily and evenly. Make sure that you never hold your breath. The breathing instructions in the photos below are a reminder of how you should be breathing when you move into the pose.

Whether you are performing Beginner Sun Salutation as a warm-up or on its own, you should perform four cycles per practice and work up to performing twelve cycles per practice. A cycle includes moving through all the poses for both sides of your body.

Beginner Sun Salutation involves a fluid motion from one pose to the next. You do not need to hold each pose.

BEGINNER SUN SALUTATION

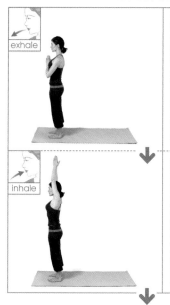

exhale

1 Begin in Mountain Pose. For information on Mountain Pose, see page 120.

• Make sure your feet are no wider than hip width apart.

2 Position your hands in Prayer Pose. For information on Prayer Pose, see page 48.

inhale

3 Circle your arms out to each side and bring your palms together overhead.

4 Press the soles of your feet into the floor and the crown of your head toward the ceiling to lengthen your spine.

BEGINNER SUN SALUTATION (CONTINUED)

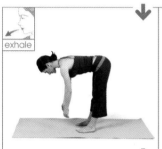

exhale

5 Bend forward from your hips until your upper body is parallel with the floor.

- Make sure you keep your back flat and your head and neck in line with your spine.

6 Let your arms dangle straight down from your shoulders.

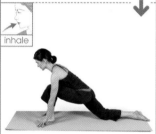

inhale

7 Bring your hands and knees to the floor and move into Table Pose.

- For information on Table Pose, see page 172.

8 Step your left foot forward between your hands and move into Lunge Pose.

- For information on Lunge Pose, see page 180.
- Make sure your left knee is directly above your left ankle.

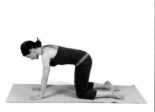

9 Bring your left knee back beside your right knee and move into Table Pose.

- Your legs should be hip width apart and your knees should be directly below your hips.

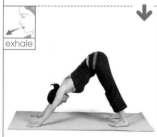

exhale

10 Tuck your toes under and lift your hips up into Downward-Facing Dog Pose.

- For information on Downward-Facing Dog Pose, see page 188.

11 Return to Table Pose.

CONTINUED...

BEGINNER SUN SALUTATION (CONTINUED)

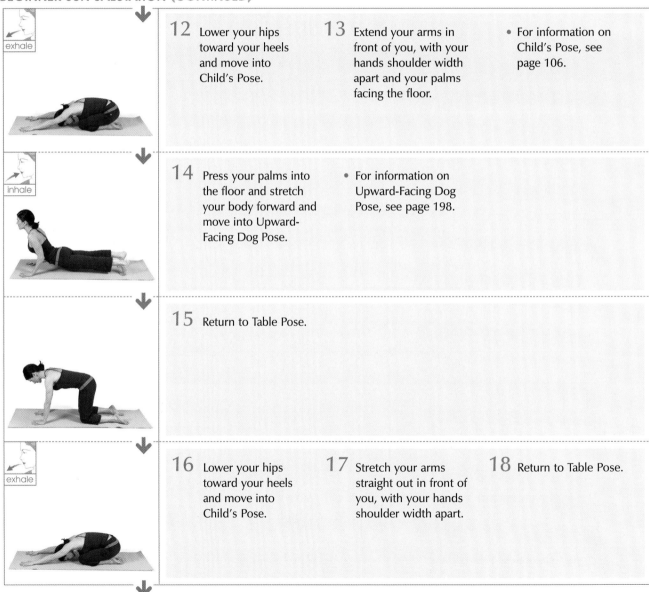

exhale

12 Lower your hips toward your heels and move into Child's Pose.

13 Extend your arms in front of you, with your hands shoulder width apart and your palms facing the floor.

- For information on Child's Pose, see page 106.

inhale

14 Press your palms into the floor and stretch your body forward and move into Upward-Facing Dog Pose.

- For information on Upward-Facing Dog Pose, see page 198.

15 Return to Table Pose.

exhale

16 Lower your hips toward your heels and move into Child's Pose.

17 Stretch your arms straight out in front of you, with your hands shoulder width apart.

18 Return to Table Pose.

BEGINNER SUN SALUTATION (CONTINUED)

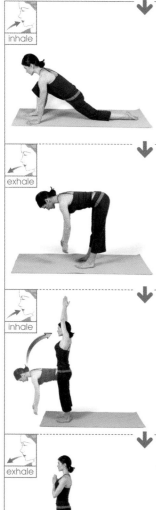

inhale

19 Step your right foot forward between your hands and move into Lunge Pose.

- Make sure your right knee is directly above your right ankle.

exhale

20 Bring your left foot forward next to your right foot.

21 Straighten your legs, lift your hips and raise your upper body until it is parallel with the floor.

- Keep your back flat and your head in line with your spine.

22 Let your arms dangle straight down from your shoulders.

inhale

23 Extend your arms beside your head, parallel to the floor.

- Your upper arms should be next to your ears and your palms should be facing in.

24 Lift your upper body to return to a standing position.

25 Stretch your arms up toward the ceiling.

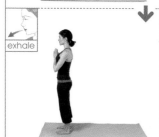

exhale

26 Lower your arms to your sides and return to Prayer Pose.

27 Repeat steps **3** to **26**, starting with your other foot in steps **8** and **19**.

sun salutation *(surya namaskar)*

Sun Salutation is a sequence of twelve yoga poses that is useful for warming up and energizing your body at the beginning of a yoga practice. This series will help to connect your body, breath and mind.

If you only have time for a quick practice, you may want to perform Sun Salutation on its own to strengthen and stretch all of your major muscle groups, while stimulating your cardiovascular system.

Each pose in this series works as a counter pose to the previous pose, allowing your spine to stretch in a different direction. As you flow from one pose to the next, focus on your body's alignment in each pose and make sure you are breathing easily. You should concentrate on learning the poses and the sequence of Sun Salutation before incorporating the breathing pattern of the series.

Whether performing Sun Salutation as a warm-up or on its own, beginners should perform four cycles per practice and work up to performing twelve cycles per practice. A cycle includes moving through all the poses for both sides of your body.

Sun Salutation involves a fluid motion from one pose to the next. You do not need to hold each pose.

SUN SALUTATION

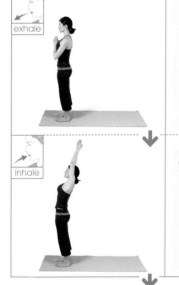

exhale

1 Begin in Mountain Pose. For information on Mountain Pose, see page 120.

- Make sure your feet are no wider than hip width apart.

2 Position your hands in Prayer Pose. For information on Prayer Pose, see page 48.

inhale

3 Circle your arms out to each side and bring your palms together overhead.

4 Move into Standing Back Bend.

- For information on Standing Back Bend, see page 192.

- Make sure you keep your spine long. Do not over-arch your lower back.

262

SUN SALUTATION (CONTINUED)

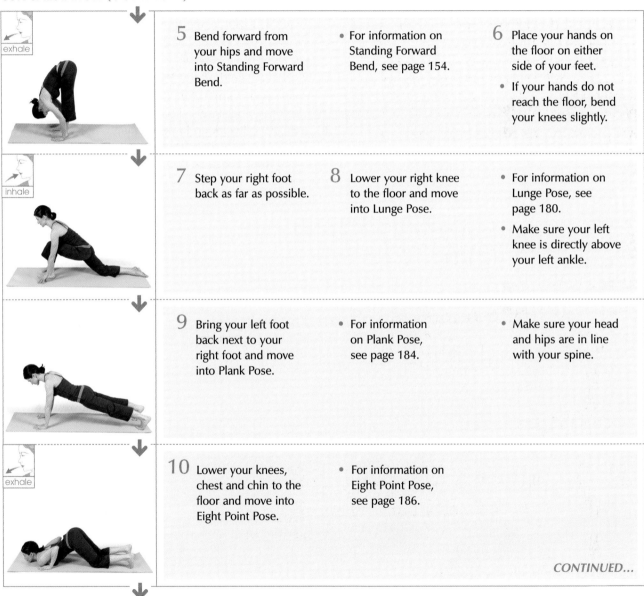

5 Bend forward from your hips and move into Standing Forward Bend.

- For information on Standing Forward Bend, see page 154.

6 Place your hands on the floor on either side of your feet.

- If your hands do not reach the floor, bend your knees slightly.

7 Step your right foot back as far as possible.

8 Lower your right knee to the floor and move into Lunge Pose.

- For information on Lunge Pose, see page 180.

- Make sure your left knee is directly above your left ankle.

9 Bring your left foot back next to your right foot and move into Plank Pose.

- For information on Plank Pose, see page 184.

- Make sure your head and hips are in line with your spine.

10 Lower your knees, chest and chin to the floor and move into Eight Point Pose.

- For information on Eight Point Pose, see page 186.

CONTINUED...

sun salutation *(surya namaskar)*

SUN SALUTATION (CONTINUED)

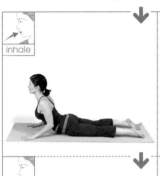

inhale

11 Slide your body forward and move into Cobra Pose.

- For information on Cobra Pose, see page 196.

- Make sure your shoulders are relaxed and down.

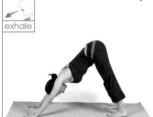

exhale

12 Tuck your toes under and lift your hips up into Downward-Facing Dog Pose.

- For information on Downward-Facing Dog Pose, see page 188.

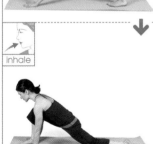

inhale

13 Step your right foot forward and place your foot between your hands.

14 Lower your left knee to the floor and move into Lunge Pose.

- Make sure your right knee is directly above your right ankle.

SUN SALUTATION (CONTINUED)

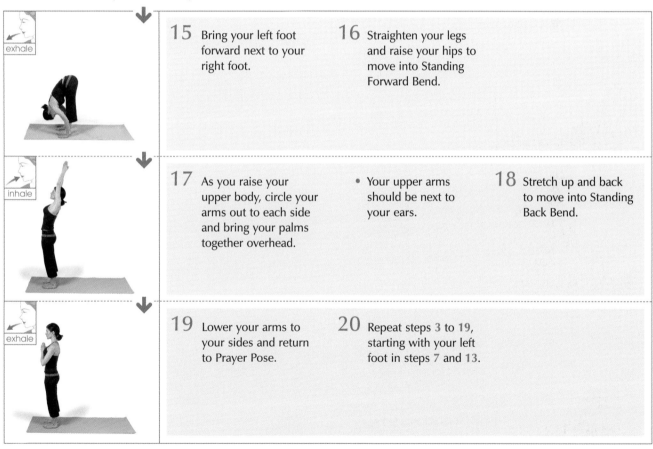

15 Bring your left foot forward next to your right foot.

16 Straighten your legs and raise your hips to move into Standing Forward Bend.

17 As you raise your upper body, circle your arms out to each side and bring your palms together overhead.

• Your upper arms should be next to your ears.

18 Stretch up and back to move into Standing Back Bend.

19 Lower your arms to your sides and return to Prayer Pose.

20 Repeat steps **3** to **19**, starting with your left foot in steps **7** and **13**.

beginner
practice 1

Beginner Practice 1 is a well-rounded practice for beginners that works your entire body. This practice moves your spine in all directions—stretching your spine forward and backward, as well as twisting your spine.

Before beginning the practice, take a few minutes to center yourself and become aware of your breathing. You should also perform a warm-up sequence, such as Seated Warm-Up Sequence shown on page 252, before you start Beginner Practice 1.

Many of the poses in this practice require you to begin in Table Pose, with your knees on the floor. If your knees are uncomfortable in this position, you can place a folded towel or blanket under them to help relieve the discomfort.

After completing the practice, you should spend 5 to 15 minutes in a relaxation or restorative pose, such as Relaxation Pose shown on page 242. Beginner Practice 1 should take approximately 30 to 45 minutes to complete, in addition to the time you take to center yourself, warm up and relax.

BEGINNER PRACTICE 1

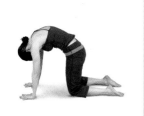

1 Begin in Table Pose. For information on Table Pose, see page 172.

- Make sure your wrists are below your shoulders and your knees are below your hips.

2 Perform Cat Stretch to improve the flexibility of your spine and the circulation in your body.

- For information on Cat Stretch, see page 174.

3 Return to Table Pose.

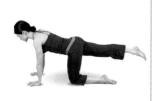

4 Move into Extended Cat Stretch.

- For information on Extended Cat Stretch, see page 176.

- Extended Cat Stretch helps stretch and warm up your spine. This pose is also beneficial for stretching your legs and neck.

5 Perform Extended Cat Stretch for your other side and then return to Table Pose.

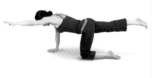

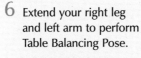

6 Extend your right leg and left arm to perform Table Balancing Pose.

- For information on Table Balancing Pose, see page 178.

- Table Balancing Pose is an energizing pose that helps improve your balance and strengthen your entire body.

7 Perform Table Balancing Pose for your other side and then return to Table Pose.

BEGINNER PRACTICE 1 (CONTINUED)

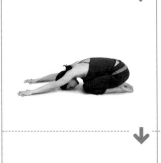

8 Lower your hips toward your heels and move into Child's Pose.

- For information on Child's Pose, see page 106.

9 Remain in Child's Pose until you feel rested and ready to continue with your practice. Then return to Table Pose.

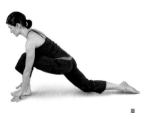

10 Step your left foot forward between your hands and move into Lunge Pose.

- For information on Lunge Pose, see page 180.
- Make sure your left knee is directly above your left ankle.

11 Perform Lunge Pose for your other side and then return to Table Pose.

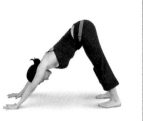

12 Tuck your toes under and lift your hips up into Downward-Facing Dog Pose.

- For information on Downward-Facing Dog Pose, see page 188.

- This pose lengthens your spine and provides an intense stretch to the back of your legs.

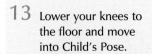

13 Lower your knees to the floor and move into Child's Pose.

14 Stretch your arms straight out in front of you, with your hands shoulder width apart.

- Feel your spine lengthen as you drop the weight of your hips toward your heels and relax your head to the floor.

CONTINUED...

beginner practice 1

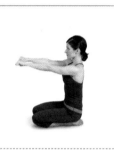

15 Lift your torso to move into Thunderbolt Pose. For information on Thunderbolt Pose, see page 90.

16 Raise both arms to shoulder height in front of you.

17 Make fists with your hands and then rotate your wrists 3 to 5 times in each direction.

- These wrist rotations help relieve tension in your wrists.

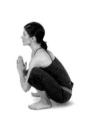

18 Place the soles of your feet on the floor, hip width apart and move into Squat Pose.

- For information on Squat Pose, see page 68.

- Squat Pose helps open your hips, groin and inner thighs, while stretching your ankles and feet.

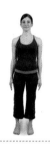

19 Lift your hips and then perform Spinal Roll to roll your spine up one vertebra at a time.

- For information on Spinal Roll, see page 49.

20 Move into Mountain Pose.

- For information on Mountain Pose, see page 120.

- Mountain Pose can improve your posture, stability and balance.

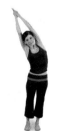

21 Bring your palms together over your head and move into Crescent Moon Pose.

- For information on Crescent Moon Pose, see page 124.

- Crescent Moon Pose is an energizing pose that opens and stretches the sides of your body.

22 Perform Crescent Moon Pose for your other side and then return to Mountain Pose.

BEGINNER PRACTICE 1 (CONTINUED)

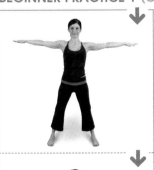

23 Step your right foot to the right 3 to 5 feet and move into Five Pointed Star Pose.

- For information on Five Pointed Star Pose, see page 122.

- Five Pointed Star Pose energizes and lengthens your entire body.

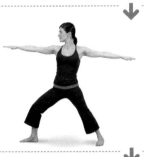

24 Turn your right foot out 90 degrees and then turn your left foot in 45 degrees and move into Warrior II Pose.

- For information on Warrior II Pose, see page 130.
- Warrior II Pose strengthens and stretches your legs, ankles, shoulders and arms.

25 Perform Warrior II Pose for your other side and then return to Mountain Pose.

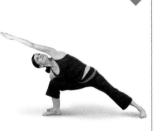

26 Step your right foot to the right approximately 3 feet and move into Side Angle Pose.

- For information on Side Angle Pose, see page 132.

- Side Angle Pose provides an intense stretch along the sides of your body, especially the sides of your waist and rib cage.

27 Perform Side Angle Pose for your other side and then return to Mountain Pose.

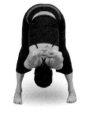

28 Position your feet slightly wider than hip width apart and interlace your fingers behind your back.

29 Perform Standing Yoga Mudra Pose.

- For information on Standing Yoga Mudra Pose, see page 166.

- This pose stretches your shoulders, upper back and legs and helps increase the flexibility of your spine and hips.

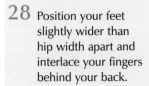

beginner practice 2

Beginner Practice 2 is a well-rounded beginner practice that ensures you work your entire body. This practice incorporates the three basic movements of the spine—forward bends, back bends and twists.

Before you start Beginner Practice 2, you should take a few minutes to center yourself and become aware of your breathing. You should then perform a warm-up sequence, such as Seated Warm-Up Sequence, which is shown on page 252.

After the practice, you should take 5 to 15 minutes to perform a relaxation pose. Relaxing at the end of the practice allows released energy to flow through your body.

Beginner Practice 2 will take 30 to 40 minutes to complete, not including the time you spend centering, warming up and relaxing. The length of the practice depends on how long you hold the poses and the time you take to move from one pose to the next.

BEGINNER PRACTICE 2

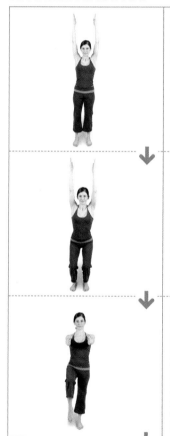

1 Begin in Mountain Pose.

- For information on Mountain Pose, see page 120.

2 Raise your arms above your head, keeping your shoulders relaxed and down.

- Your arms should be shoulder width apart and your palms should be facing each other.

- This modification of Mountain Pose stretches your arms and shoulders.

3 Keeping your arms above your head, bend your knees and move into Chair Pose.

- For information on Chair Pose, see page 126.

- Chair Pose strengthens your lower body and torso.

4 Return to Mountain Pose.

5 Bend your right leg and bring your right knee up until your thigh is parallel to the floor and move into Stork Pose.

- For information on Stork Pose, see page 138.

- Stork Pose is a balancing pose that helps to open your hips and strengthen your legs, arms and shoulders.

6 Perform Stork Pose for your other side and then return to Mountain Pose.

BEGINNER PRACTICE 2 (CONTINUED)

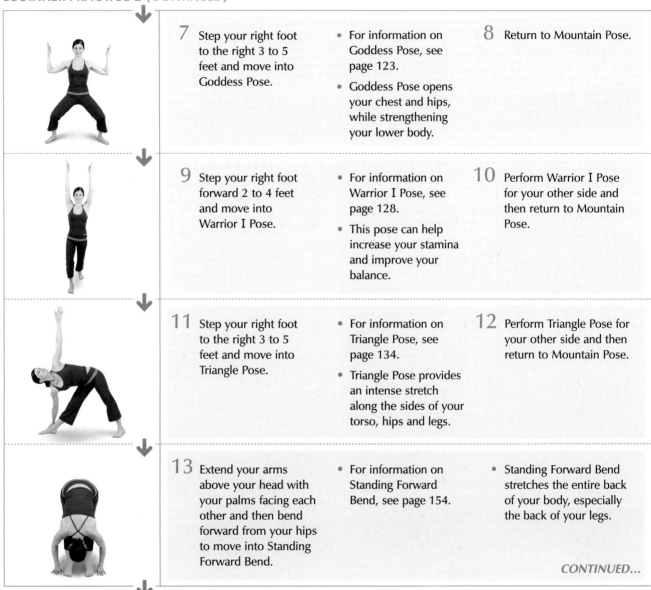

7 Step your right foot to the right 3 to 5 feet and move into Goddess Pose.

- For information on Goddess Pose, see page 123.
- Goddess Pose opens your chest and hips, while strengthening your lower body.

8 Return to Mountain Pose.

9 Step your right foot forward 2 to 4 feet and move into Warrior I Pose.

- For information on Warrior I Pose, see page 128.
- This pose can help increase your stamina and improve your balance.

10 Perform Warrior I Pose for your other side and then return to Mountain Pose.

11 Step your right foot to the right 3 to 5 feet and move into Triangle Pose.

- For information on Triangle Pose, see page 134.
- Triangle Pose provides an intense stretch along the sides of your torso, hips and legs.

12 Perform Triangle Pose for your other side and then return to Mountain Pose.

13 Extend your arms above your head with your palms facing each other and then bend forward from your hips to move into Standing Forward Bend.

- For information on Standing Forward Bend, see page 154.

- Standing Forward Bend stretches the entire back of your body, especially the back of your legs.

CONTINUED...

beginner practice 2

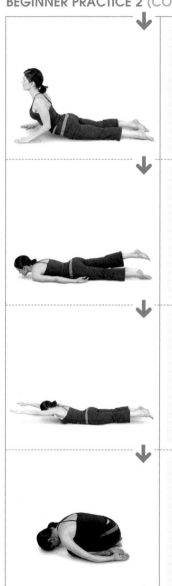

14 Lie face-down on the floor with your legs no wider than hip width apart and your palms on the floor under your shoulders.

15 Slowly curl your spine up to move into Cobra Pose.

- For information on Cobra Pose, see page 196.
- Cobra Pose develops strength and flexibility in your spine and lower back.

16 Lie face-down on the floor, place your arms on the floor alongside your body and rest your chin on the floor.

17 Lift your right leg toward the ceiling to move into Half Locust Pose.

- For information on Half Locust Pose, see page 202.

- Half Locust Pose is beneficial for strengthening your legs and lower back.

18 Perform Half Locust Pose for your other side.

19 Lie face-down on the floor, stretch your arms straight in front of you, with your palms facing down and rest your forehead on the floor.

20 Lift your arms, chest, head and both legs up to move into Front Lying Boat Pose.

- For information on Front Lying Boat Pose, see page 200.

- Front Lying Boat Pose strengthens your back and helps to develop your stamina and concentration.

21 Place your hands under your shoulders and lift your body up and back into Child's Pose.

- For information on Child's Pose, see page 106.

- Child's Pose is a good counter pose for back bends and will help release tension from your lower back.

22 Remain in Child's Pose until you feel rested and ready to continue with your practice.

BEGINNER PRACTICE 2 (CONTINUED)

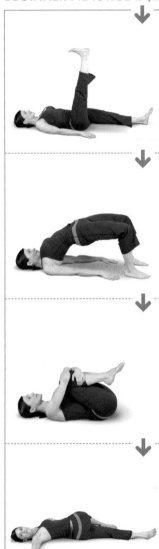

23 Lie on your back on the floor with your legs extended, your feet together and your arms at your sides.

24 Flex your right foot and lift your right leg toward the ceiling to perform Leg Raises.

- For information on Leg Raises, see page 54.

- Leg Raises strengthen your abdominals and lower back.

25 Perform Leg Raises for your other side.

26 Lying on your back, bend your knees and place your feet flat on the floor, hip width apart.

27 Lift your pelvis off the floor to move into Bridge Pose.

- For information on Bridge Pose, see page 208.

- Bridge Pose increases the flexibility of your spine and stretches your neck, abdomen and thighs.

28 Lying on your back, bend your knees and place your feet flat on the floor, hip width apart.

29 Draw your knees toward your chest to move into Little Boat Pose.

- For information on Little Boat Pose, see page 58.

- Little Boat Pose stretches and releases your spine, lower back and hips and is useful as a counter pose for Bridge Pose.

30 Extend your legs and place your arms out to your sides at shoulder height.

31 Place the sole of your right foot just above your left knee and then lower your right knee toward the floor on the left side of your body to perform Knee Down Twist.

- For information on Knee Down Twist, see page 236.

- Knee Down Twist opens your chest and shoulders.

chair yoga practice

Chair Yoga Practice is a yoga practice that you can perform while seated in a chair. When sitting in a chair for a long period of time, you may find your back, shoulders and neck become tense. This practice can help you relieve this tension, as well as let go of any stress.

Chair Yoga Practice is particularly useful if you need a short break from sitting or if you want to fit a yoga practice into your busy day. For example, you may want to perform this practice if you sit in a chair at work all day or if you are traveling on a plane or train. Chair Yoga Practice is also useful for seniors and people who have trouble sitting on the floor.

Before you begin, you should take a few minutes to focus on breathing and centering yourself and then perform the warm-up shown below. The entire warm-up and practice should take 20 to 30 minutes.

CHAIR YOGA WARM-UP

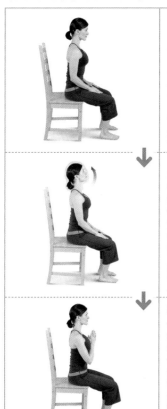

1 Begin in Seated Mountain Pose.

• For information on Seated Mountain Pose, see page 110.

2 Press your sitting bones into the seat of the chair and point the crown of your head toward the ceiling to lengthen your spine.

3 Perform neck stretches to relax your head and warm up your neck.

• For information on neck stretches, see page 42.

4 Bring your palms together in front of your chest in Prayer Pose.

• For information on Prayer Pose, see page 48.

• Your elbows should be lower than your wrists and your fingers should be pointing toward the ceiling.

• Prayer Pose can help to increase the flexibility of your wrists.

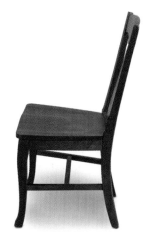
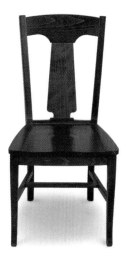
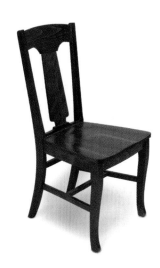

CHAIR YOGA WARM-UP (CONTINUED)

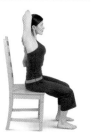

5 Circle your arms out to each side and then bring your palms together overhead to perform arm stretches.

• For information on arm stretches, see page 46.

• Arm stretches improve the circulation in your upper body, including your arms, hands, fingers and the area around your heart.

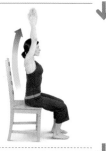

6 Bend your left elbow and bring your left forearm behind your back, resting the back of your hand in the middle of your back, near your shoulder blades.

7 Extend your right arm over your head. Then bend your right elbow and clasp the fingers of your left hand with your right hand.

8 Repeat steps 6 and 7 for your other side and then return to Seated Mountain Pose.

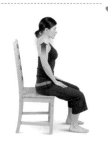

9 Perform shoulder stretches to relieve tightness in your upper back, shoulders and neck.

• For information on shoulder stretches, see page 44.

CONTINUED...

275

chair yoga practice

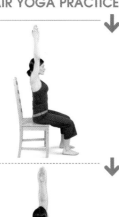

10 Raise your arms above your head, keeping your shoulders relaxed and down.

- Your arms should be shoulder width apart and your palms should be facing each other.

- This Seated Mountain Pose modification stretches your arms and shoulders and increases circulation in your upper body.

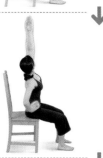

11 Place your right hand on your right hip and extend your left arm overhead, with your palm facing in.

12 Stretch to the right to perform Seated Side Bend.

- For information on Seated Side Bend, see page 82.

- Seated Side Bend stretches the sides of your body, from your hips to your fingertips.

13 Perform steps **11** and **12** for your other side and then return to Seated Mountain Pose.

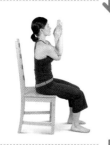

14 Raise your arms to shoulder height in front of you, palms facing up.

15 Cross your left arm over your right arm so your elbows are on top of each other.

16 Bend your elbows and wrap your forearms around each other so your palms are facing each other, with your fingers pointing toward the ceiling.

17 Repeat steps **14** to **16** for your other side and then return to Seated Mountain Pose.

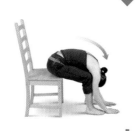

18 Extend your arms over your head and then bend forward from your hips to move into Chair Forward Bend.

- For information on Chair Forward Bend, see page 114.

- Chair Forward Bend soothes your nervous system and encourages your mind to release stress.

19 Return to Seated Mountain Pose.

CHAIR YOGA PRACTICE (CONTINUED)

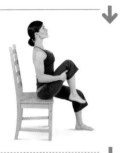

20 Interlace your fingers under your right thigh and lift your right knee up toward your chest to move into Seated Knee to Chest Pose.

- For information on Seated Knee to Chest Pose, see page 113.
- Seated Knee to Chest Pose stretches your hips and thighs while strengthening your back.

21 Perform Seated Knee to Chest Pose for your other side and then return to Seated Mountain Pose.

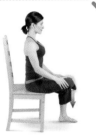

22 Place your right ankle on top of your left knee and rest your right hand just above your right knee.

23 Gently press your right knee toward the floor to perform Chair Hip Stretch.

- For information on Chair Hip Stretch, see page 112.

- Chair Hip Stretch stretches and opens your hips.

24 Perform Chair Hip Stretch for your other side and then return to Seated Mountain Pose.

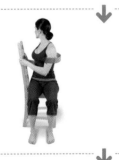

25 Position the right side of your body facing the chair back and hold the chair back with your hands at approximately shoulder height.

26 Twist to the right to move into Chair Twist.

- For information on Chair Twist, see page 116.

- Chair Twist relieves stiffness in your neck, shoulders and upper back.

27 Perform Chair Twist for your other side and then return to Seated Mountain Pose.

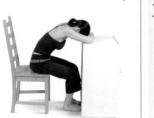

28 Position your chair close to a table and perform Chair Forward Bend, resting your forearms on the table and resting your head on your forearms.

29 Stay in this pose for 1 to 5 minutes and allow your body to relax. Observe and become aware of your breath as you hold the pose.

relaxation practice

The sequence of poses in Relaxation Practice will help to relax your body and mind. You may want to perform this practice just before you go to bed to release any stress you may be feeling and prepare yourself for sleep. Performing Relaxation Practice may lower your body temperature, so you may want to wear an extra layer of clothing.

Before you begin Relaxation Practice, you should perform Reclined Warm-Up Sequence shown on page 254. You should also take a few minutes to

concentrate on your breathing and centering yourself before you begin.

To perform Relaxation Practice, you will need three blankets and a bolster. Make sure these props are readily accessible so you do not need to go searching for them during the middle of your practice.

After you complete Relaxation Practice, you should spend 5 to 15 minutes in Relaxation Pose as shown on page 242.

RELAXATION PRACTICE

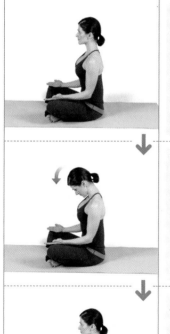

1 Begin in Easy Pose.

• For information on Easy Pose, see page 74.

2 Press your sitting bones toward the floor and point the crown of your head toward the ceiling to lengthen your spine.

3 Perform neck stretches to relax your head and warm up your neck.

• For information on neck stretches, see page 42.

4 Perform shoulder stretches to relieve tightness and tension in your upper back and shoulders.

• For information on shoulder stretches, see page 44.

RELAXATION PRACTICE (CONTINUED)

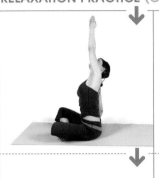

5 Place your right palm on the floor beside your right hip and raise your left arm overhead.

6 Stretch to the right to move into Seated Side Bend and stretch the side of your body.

- For information on Seated Side Bend, see page 82.

7 Perform Seated Side Bend for your other side and then return to Easy Pose.

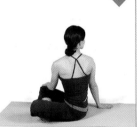

8 Turn your upper body toward the right and move into Simple Twist.

- For information on Simple Twist, see page 84.
- Simple Twist helps to increase the flexibility of your spine and upper back.

9 Perform Simple Twist for your other side and then return to Easy Pose.

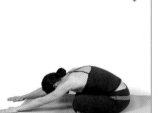

10 Bend forward from your hips and move into Easy Pose Forward Bend.

- For information on Easy Pose Forward Bend, see page 96.

- Easy Pose Forward Bend can soothe your nervous system, which helps clear and calm your mind.

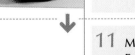

11 Move into Table Pose. For information on Table Pose, see page 172.

- Make sure your wrists are below your shoulders and your knees are below your hips.

12 Perform Cat Stretch to improve the flexibility of and circulation in your spine.

- For information on Cat Stretch, see page 174.

13 Return to Table Pose.

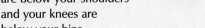

CONTINUED...

relaxation practice

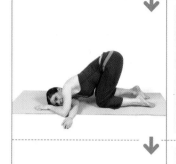

14 Slide your right arm under your body to move into Thread the Needle Pose.

• For information on Thread the Needle Pose, see page 182.

15 Perform Thread the Needle Pose for your other side.

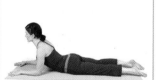

16 Lie face down with your legs extended behind you and your feet hip width apart.

17 Place your elbows directly under your shoulders with your forearms flat on the floor and then move into Sphinx Pose.

• For information on Sphinx Pose, see page 194.

• This pose is useful for calming your nervous system.

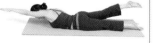

18 Extend your left arm in front of you and your right arm at your side, palms down and your forehead on the floor.

19 Raise your left arm, your chest, head and right leg off the floor to perform a modified Front Lying Boat Pose.

• For information on Front Lying Boat Pose, see page 200.

20 Repeat the modification for your other arm and leg.

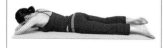

21 Rest the top of your feet on the floor with your toes pointing outward.

22 Cross your arms in front of your head to move into Crocodile Pose.

• For information on Crocodile Pose, see page 244.

• Crocodile Pose is useful for relieving stress and tension in your body. You should feel calm and rejuvenated after performing Crocodile Pose.

RELAXATION PRACTICE (CONTINUED)

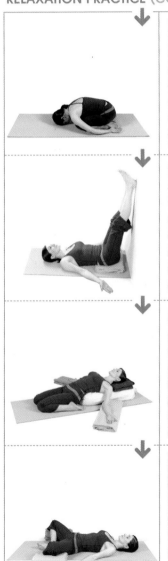

23 Place your hands under your shoulders and lift your body up and back into Child's Pose.

- For information on Child's Pose, see page 106.

- A bolster can make this pose more relaxing. Place a bolster between your knees and then rest your upper body, arms and head on the bolster.

24 Sit on a folded blanket approximately 3 inches away from a wall, with your legs extended and your right side facing the wall.

25 Lower your upper body to the floor as you move into Legs Up the Wall Pose.

- For information on Legs Up the Wall Pose, see page 218.

- Legs Up the Wall Pose helps reduce tension in your head, neck and shoulders.

26 Place a folded blanket on top of one end of a bolster on the floor. Then position folded blankets on either side of the bolster.

27 Sit in Hero Pose in front of the bolster and then lean back onto the bolster to perform Supported Reclining Hero Pose.

- For information on Supported Reclining Hero Pose, see page 246.

- This pose helps soothe your mind and relax your nervous system.

28 Lie on your back on the floor with your knees bent and the soles of your feet flat on the floor.

29 Bring the soles of your feet together and allow your knees to drop toward the floor to move into Reclined Bound Angle Pose.

30 Place folded blankets under each thigh to support your knees.

- For information on Reclined Bound Angle Pose, see page 238.

stress management practice

Stress Management Practice includes a sequence of poses that help your mind and body release stress and tension.

You should take 5 to 10 minutes before you begin the practice to center yourself and become aware of your breathing. Becoming aware of your breath and body are important for reducing stress. You should then perform Reclined Warm-Up Sequence shown on page 254.

STRESS MANAGEMENT PRACTICE

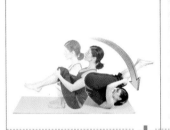

1 Sit on the floor with your knees bent, as close to your chest as possible and hold your legs just below or behind your knees.

2 Round your spine and roll backward to perform Spinal Rocking.

- For information on Spinal Rocking, see page 50.
- Spinal Rocking massages your spine, which helps relax your nervous system.

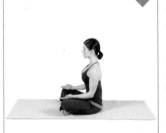

3 Sit on the floor with your legs crossed in front of you and move into Easy Pose.

- For information on Easy Pose, see page 74.
- Easy Pose is a calming pose that is useful for meditation.

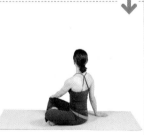

4 Turn your upper body toward the right and move into Simple Twist.

- For information on Simple Twist, see page 84.
- Simple Twist is useful for stretching your spine, shoulders and upper chest.

5 Perform Simple Twist for your other side.

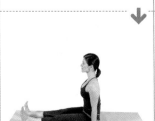

6 Extend your legs in front of you and move into Staff Pose.

- For information on Staff Pose, see page 72.
- Staff Pose can help improve your posture.

STRESS MANAGEMENT PRACTICE (CONTINUED)

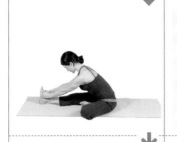

7 Bend your left leg and place the sole of your left foot against the inside of your right thigh.

8 Extend your arms overhead and bend forward from your hips to move into Head to Knee Pose.

- For information on Head to Knee Pose, see page 98.

- Head to Knee Pose provides an intense stretch to the back of your legs.

9 Perform Head to Knee Pose for your other side.

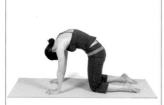

10 Move into Table Pose. For information on Table Pose, see page 172.

- Make sure your wrists are directly below your shoulders and your knees are directly below your hips.

11 Perform Cat Stretch to improve the flexibility of your spine and release tension from your body.

- For information on Cat Stretch, see page 174.

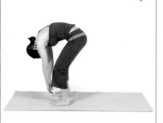

12 Move into Squat Pose. For information on Squat Pose, see page 68.

13 Place your hands on the floor slightly in front of you, with your palms facing down and lift your hips toward the ceiling.

14 Tuck your tailbone under and slowly roll your spine up.

- For information on Spinal Roll, see page 49.

- Spinal Roll can relieve tension in your spine.

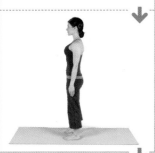

15 Stand tall and relaxed with your feet hip width apart in Mountain Pose.

- For information on Mountain Pose, see page 120.

- Take time to relax, remain still and breathe evenly in this pose.

CONTINUED...

stress management
practice

At the end of the practice, you should take 5 to 15 minutes to perform Relaxation Pose. This provides you with an opportunity to further relax and meditate.

Stress Management Practice should take 30 to 45 minutes, not including the time you spend centering, warming up and relaxing. To ensure you remain relaxed, do not rush through the practice. You should move slowly from one pose to the next.

STRESS MANAGEMENT PRACTICE (CONTINUED)

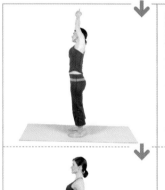

16 Circle your arms out to each side, then bring your palms together overhead and move into Crescent Moon Pose.

- For information on Crescent Moon Pose, see page 124.
- Crescent Moon Pose is an energizing pose that opens and stretches the sides of your body.

17 Perform Crescent Moon Pose for your other side and then return to Mountain Pose.

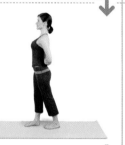

18 Step your right foot forward and clasp your elbows behind your back.

19 Lift your chest forward and gently arch your spine.

- This variation of Standing Back Bend opens your chest and stretches the front of your body.
- For information on Standing Back Bend, see page 192.

20 Repeat this variation with your other foot forward and then return to Mountain Pose.

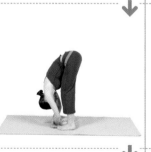

21 Step your right foot to the right 2 to 3 feet and then bend forward from your hips, bending your knees slightly.

22 Relax your head and neck toward the floor and move into Rag Doll Pose.

- For information on Rag Doll Pose, see page 168.

- Rag Doll Pose is beneficial for relieving tension in your head, neck, shoulders and lower back.

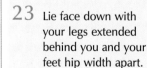

23 Lie face down with your legs extended behind you and your feet hip width apart.

24 Place your elbows directly under your shoulders with your forearms flat on the floor and move into Sphinx Pose.

- For information on Sphinx Pose, see page 194.
- This pose is useful for calming your nervous system.

STRESS MANAGEMENT PRACTICE (CONTINUED)

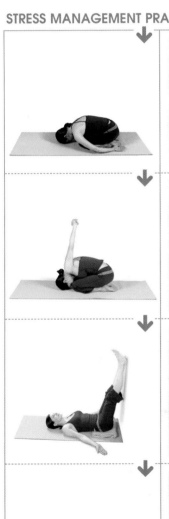

25 Place your hands under your shoulders and lift your body up and back into Child's Pose.

- For information on Child's Pose, see page 106.

- Breathe evenly while performing this pose and visualize your body softening with each breath.

26 Kneel on the floor with your knees hip width apart and sit back onto your heels.

27 Interlace your fingers behind your back, bend forward and move into Seated Yoga Mudra Pose.

- For information on Seated Yoga Mudra Pose, see page 104.

- Seated Yoga Mudra Pose clears your mind and reconnects your heart and mind.

28 Sit on a folded blanket approximately 3 inches away from a wall, with your legs extended and your right side facing the wall.

29 Lower your upper body to the floor as you move into Legs Up the Wall Pose.

- For information on Legs Up the Wall Pose, see page 218.

- Legs Up the Wall Pose helps reduce tension in your head, neck and shoulders.

30 Lie on your back with your legs extended and your arms out to your sides at shoulder height.

31 Place the sole of your right foot just above your left knee and then lower your right knee toward the floor on the left side of your body to perform Knee Down Twist.

- For information on Knee Down Twist, see page 236.

32 Repeat Knee Down Twist for your other side.

intermediate practice

Intermediate Practice is a more intense and challenging yoga practice you can perform when you are comfortable with the beginner practices.

Before beginning Intermediate Practice, make sure you take a few moments to center yourself and become aware of your breath. You should then perform a warm-up sequence, such as the sequence shown on page 252 or 256. You can also create your own warm-up sequence by performing any of the poses described in the Warm-Up Poses chapter of this book on pages 42 to 69.

INTERMEDIATE PRACTICE

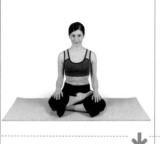

1 Begin in Staff Pose. For information on Staff Pose, see page 72.

2 Bend your right leg, place your right foot on your left thigh and move into Half Lotus Pose.

- For information on Half Lotus Pose, see page 78.

- To warm up for Half Lotus Pose, you can perform Rock the Baby, as shown on page 52.

3 Perform Half Lotus Pose for your other side and then return to Staff Pose.

4 Bend your left leg and bring your left heel under your right thigh. Then bend your right leg over your left knee and move into Cow Face Pose.

- For information on Cow Face Pose, see page 80.

- Cow Face Pose provides a good stretch for your arms and shoulders.

5 Perform Cow Face Pose for your other side and then return to Staff Pose.

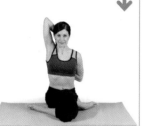

6 Kneel on the floor with your knees hip width apart and extend your right leg to your right side to move into Gate Pose.

- For information on Gate Pose, see page 64.

- Gate Pose stretches the sides of your body and increases the flexibility of your spine.

7 Perform Gate Pose for your other side and then move into Mountain Pose. For information on Mountain Pose, see page 120.

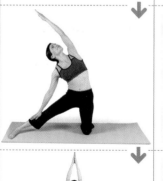

8 Bend your right leg, placing the sole of your right foot against the inside of your left leg to move into Tree Pose.

- For information on Tree Pose, see page 142.

- Tree Pose can strengthen your legs, ankles and feet and help increase the flexibility of your hips and knees.

9 Perform Tree Pose for your other side and then return to Mountain Pose.

INTERMEDIATE PRACTICE (CONTINUED)

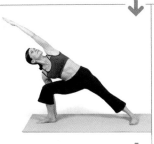

10 Step your right foot to the right approximately 3 feet and then move into Side Angle Pose.

- For information on Side Angle Pose, see page 132.

- Side Angle Pose provides an intense stretch along the sides of your body, especially the sides of your waist and rib cage.

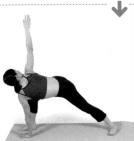

11 Move into Side Angle Twist.

- For information on Side Angle Twist, see page 160.

- Side Angle Twist is useful for improving your balance and strengthening your legs and torso.

12 Perform Side Angle Pose and Side Angle Twist for your other side and then return to Mountain Pose.

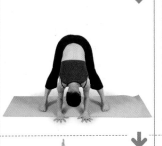

13 Step your right foot to the right 2 to 3 feet and place your hands on your hips.

14 Bend forward and move into Standing Wide Angle Forward Bend.

- For information on Standing Wide Angle Forward Bend, see page 156.

- Standing Wide Angle Forward Bend stretches the back of your legs and your inner thighs.

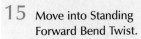

15 Move into Standing Forward Bend Twist.

- For information on Standing Forward Bend Twist, see page 158.

- This pose is beneficial for toning your abdominal muscles, releasing tension in your upper body and improving your circulation.

16 Perform Standing Forward Bend Twist for your other side.

CONTINUED...

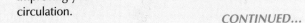

intermediate practice

Intermediate Practice should take approximately 45 to 60 minutes to complete, in addition to the time you spend centering yourself, warming up and relaxing. The length of the practice will depend on how long you hold the poses and the time you take to move from one pose to the next.

After you have completed the practice, you should take 5 to 15 minutes to perform Relaxation Pose, as shown on page 242, and allow yourself to connect with the natural flow of your breath.

INTERMEDIATE PRACTICE (CONTINUED)

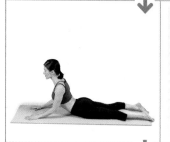

17 Lie face-down on the floor with your legs no wider than hip width apart and your palms on the floor under your shoulders.

18 Slowly curl your spine up to move into Cobra Pose.

- For information on Cobra Pose, see page 196.

- Cobra Pose develops strength and flexibility in your spine and lower back.

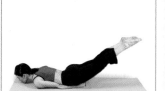

19 Lying face-down on the floor, place your arms on the floor alongside your body with your palms down and rest your chin on the floor.

20 Perform Locust Pose.

- For information on Locust Pose, see page 204.

- Locust Pose is beneficial for strengthening your legs and lower back.

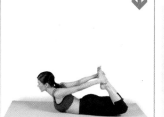

21 Lying face-down on the floor, bend your knees as you reach back with your hands and clasp your ankles or the top of your feet and move into Bow Pose.

- For information on Bow Pose, see page 206.

- Bow Pose increases the strength and flexibility of your spine, opens your chest and stimulates your abdominal area.

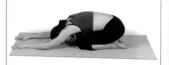

22 Place your hands under your shoulders and lift your body up and back into Child's Pose.

- For information on Child's Pose, see page 106.

- Child's Pose is a good counter pose for back bends and will help release tension from your lower back.

23 Remain in Child's Pose until you feel rested and ready to continue with your practice. Then return to Staff Pose.

INTERMEDIATE PRACTICE (CONTINUED)

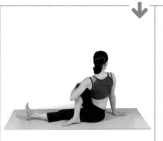

24 Bend your right knee, place your right foot on the floor outside your left thigh and move into Seated Half Spinal Twist.

- For information on Seated Half Spinal Twist, see page 86.

- Seated Half Spinal Twist is a stimulating pose that helps increase the flexibility of your spine.

25 Perform Seated Half Spinal Twist for your other side.

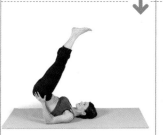

26 Lie on your back with your knees bent, the soles of your feet flat on the floor and your arms alongside your body with your palms down.

27 Draw your knees toward your chest and move into Half Shoulderstand.

- For information on Half Shoulderstand, see page 220.

- This pose is beneficial for strengthening your entire body and improving your circulation.

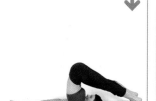

28 Slowly lower your feet toward the floor behind your head to move into Plow Pose.

- For information on Plow Pose, see page 224.

- Plow Pose stretches the entire back of your body and stimulates your nervous system.

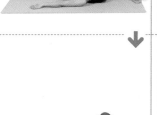

29 Lie on your back with your legs extended and your feet together. Your arms should be straight and your palms should be on the floor underneath you.

30 Press your elbows into the floor and move into Fish Pose.

- For information on Fish Pose, see page 210.

- Fish Pose is a good counter pose for Half Shoulderstand and Plow Pose because the pose stretches your neck in the opposite direction.

strengthening practice

You can perform Strengthening Practice to help build strength in your entire body. This practice also helps you build strong bones and overall flexibility.

Before you begin the practice, you should take 5 to 10 minutes to center yourself and become aware of your breath from a seated or reclined position. Then perform a standing warm-up sequence, such as Standing Warm-Up Sequence shown on page 256, to energize and help prepare your body for the poses in Strengthening Practice.

STRENGTHENING PRACTICE

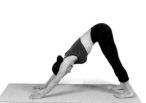

1 Begin in Table Pose. For information on Table Pose, see page 172.

2 Slide your right knee forward between your hands and move into Pigeon Pose.

- For information on Pigeon Pose, see page 66.
- Pigeon Pose helps increase the flexibility of your hips and groin, strengthen your back and stretch your thighs.

3 Perform Pigeon Pose for your other side and then return to Table Pose.

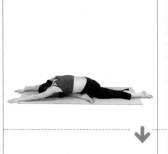

4 Tuck your toes under and lift your hips up into Downward-Facing Dog Pose.

- For information on Downward-Facing Dog Pose, see page 188.
- Downward-Facing Dog Pose lengthens your spine and stretches the back of your legs.

5 Lower your knees to the floor to return to Table Pose.

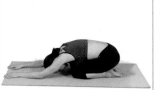

6 Lower your hips toward your heels and move into Child's Pose.

7 Extend your arms in front of you, with your hands shoulder width apart and your palms facing the floor.

- For information on Child's Pose, see page 106.
- This modification of Child's Pose stretches your shoulders, back and hips.

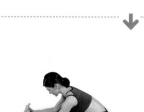

8 Begin in Staff Pose. For information on Staff Pose, see page 72.

9 Extend your arms overhead and then bend forward from your hips to move into Seated Forward Bend.

- For information on Seated Forward Bend, see page 100.

- Seated Forward Bend provides an intense stretch to the back of your body.

10 Return to Staff Pose.

STRENGTHENING PRACTICE (CONTINUED)

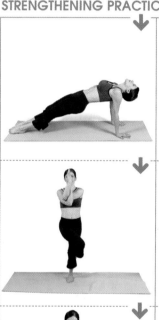

11 Place your palms on the floor behind your hips, shoulder width apart, with your fingers pointing away from you.

12 Lift your hips toward the ceiling and move into Inclined Plane Pose.

- For information on Inclined Plane Pose, see page 212.

- Inclined Plane Pose strengthens your arms, wrists and upper body.

13 Move into Mountain Pose. For information on Mountain Pose, see page 120.

14 Cross your arms and legs in Eagle Pose.

- For information on Eagle Pose, see page 146.

- Eagle Pose helps improve your balance and strengthen your legs, knees and ankles.

15 Perform Eagle Pose for your other side and then return to Mountain Pose.

16 Bend your right knee and bring your right leg behind you.

17 Reach behind you with your right hand to clasp your right ankle and move into Dancer Pose.

- For information on Dancer Pose, see page 140.

- Dancer Pose helps strengthen your shoulders, arms and legs.

18 Perform Dancer Pose for your other side and then return to Mountain Pose.

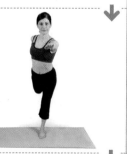

19 Step your right foot to the right 3 to 5 feet and move into Triangle Pose.

- For information on Triangle Pose, see page 134.

- Triangle Pose helps increase the strength and flexibility of your legs and stretches the sides of your body.

20 Perform Triangle Pose for your other side and then return to Mountain Pose.

CONTINUED...

strengthening practice

Strengthening Practice should take approximately 30 to 45 minutes to complete, in addition to the time you spend centering, warming up and relaxing.

It is important to perform Little Boat Pose and Little Boat Twist at the end of this practice. These poses cool down your body to help make the transition from the strengthening poses to the relaxation portion of your practice. To relax after you have completed the poses, spend 5 to 15 minutes in Relaxation Pose shown on page 242.

STRENGTHENING PRACTICE (CONTINUED)

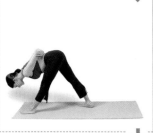

21 Clasp your elbows or wrists behind your back, step your right foot forward approximately 3 feet and move into Pyramid Pose.

- For information on Pyramid Pose, see page 162.

- Pyramid Pose helps strengthen your legs, increase the flexibility of your hips and improve your balance.

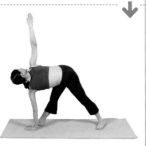

22 Move into Triangle Twist.

- For information on Triangle Twist, see page 164.

- Triangle Twist provides an intense stretch to your legs.

23 Perform Pyramid Pose and Triangle Twist for your other side and then return to Mountain Pose.

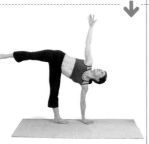

24 Bend forward from your hips and place your palms on the floor in front of your feet, shoulder width apart and then move into Half Moon Pose.

- For information on Half Moon Pose, see page 148.

- This pose can strengthen your legs and buttocks, as well as increase the flexibility of your legs and hips.

25 Perform Half Moon Pose for your other side.

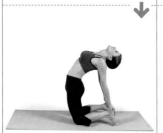

26 Kneel on the floor with your knees and feet hip width apart, curl your toes under and place your hands on your lower back, with your fingers pointing down.

27 Lift your ribcage up and back as you move into Camel Pose.

- For information on Camel Pose, see page 214.

- Camel Pose strengthens your back and spine and stretches the front of your thighs.

28 Perform Child's Pose to return your spine to a neutral position.

STRENGTHENING PRACTICE (CONTINUED)

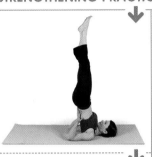

29 Lie on your back with your arms alongside your body, your legs extended and your feet together.

30 Raise both feet toward the ceiling to form a 90-degree angle with your body and legs and then move into Shoulderstand.

- For information on Shoulderstand, see page 222.
- Shoulderstand strengthens your entire body.

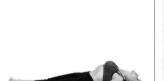

31 Lie on your back with your legs extended and your feet and legs together. Your arms should be straight and your palms should be on the floor underneath you.

32 Press your elbows into the floor to move into Fish Pose.

- For information on Fish Pose, see page 210.

- Fish Pose is a good counter pose for Shoulderstand because the pose stretches your neck in the opposite direction.

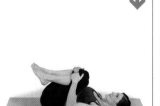

33 Lie on your back with your knees bent and your feet flat on the floor, hip width apart.

34 Draw your knees toward your chest and move into Little Boat Pose.

- For information on Little Boat Pose, see page 58.

- Little Boat Pose stretches your lower back and helps your body cool down.

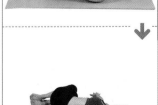

35 Extend your arms out to your sides at shoulder height, with your palms facing down.

36 Lower your knees to the right toward the floor and perform Little Boat Twist.

- For information on Little Boat Twist, see page 60.

- Little Boat Twist helps prepare you for the relaxation portion of your practice.

37 Perform Little Boat Twist for your other side.

index

index

index

index

index